blindsided

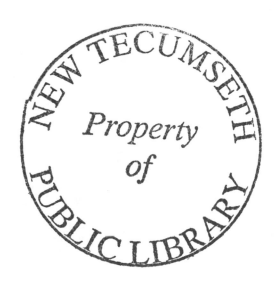
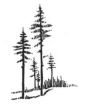

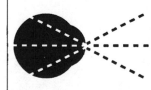

This Large Print Book carries the Seal of Approval of N.A.V.H.

blindsided

Lifting a Life Above Illness:
A Reluctant Memoir

Richard M. Cohen

Thorndike Press • Waterville, Maine

Copyright © 2004 by Richard M. Cohen.

All rights reserved.

Published in 2004 by arrangement with HarperCollins Publishers, Inc.

Thorndike Press® Large Print Biography.

The tree indicium is a trademark of Thorndike Press.

The text of this Large Print edition is unabridged.
Other aspects of the book may vary from the original edition.

Set in 16 pt. Plantin by Liana M. Walker.

Printed in the United States on permanent paper.

Library of Congress Cataloging-in-Publication Data

Cohen, Richard (Richard M.)
    Blindsided : lifting a life above illness : a reluctant memoir
/ Richard M. Cohen.
      p. cm.
    ISBN 0-7862-6654-6 (lg. print : hc : alk. paper)
  1. Cohen, Richard (Richard M.) — Health. 2. Multiple
sclerosis — Patients — Biography. 3. Large type books.
I. Title.
RC377.C544 2004b
362.1'96834'0092—dc22
   [B]   2004047926

For Meredith

And to Ben, Gabe, Lily —
our loving travel companions

Acknowledgments

"You will never write a book," my mother gently suggested a long time ago. "You work in television. That is so collaborative." She was right about the high contrast between the producer's world and a writer's quiet existence. Admittedly, it was mighty lonely in this neighborhood for the last many months. The truth, however, is that I was not on this voyage alone.

There were folks who were hugely important in the creative process. Joann Davis, my literary agent, saw the outlines and potential of this book idea before I did and stayed with it to the end, helping me to fashion and sell the book proposal. Gail Winston, a senior editor at HarperCollins, stood by the book and counseled me through many wrong turns. And Anastasia Toufexis, a freelance editor I engaged, helped guide me out of the many corners with wet paint around them.

I pay tribute to Robert Jones, editorial director at HarperCollins, who believed in this book and died only months after it was begun. Robert understood suffering and the need to cope. And how I did suffer with my own missteps.

My kids started asking when the book would be done before I fully understood what it was to be about. They kept the pressure on in difficult moments.

And of course, there was Meredith, who gave me room and kept telling me I was a better writer than I am. Please don't tell her the truth.

Cope *vb* **a:** to maintain a contest or combat usually on even terms or with success **b:** to deal with and attempt to overcome problems and difficulties.
— *Merriam-Webster's Dictionary*

That sounds simple enough.

Contents

Preface

Sometimes it seems I daydream for a living. I sit in my office on the far west side of Manhattan, trying to write but gazing out over treetops and highways to barges pushing laboriously against the current, struggling up the Hudson River. I know how that feels. The long push is relentless, and nobody has it easy. What a haul life is.

For most of any day, my face is pressed to the computer screen, my back arched and aching, stiff from sitting hour after hour in that tortured position. I assume this awkward pose because I am legally blind and must go cheek to cheek with the screen just to see it clearly enough to work.

The river traffic I casually watch moves in exquisite detail only in my mind's eye. Little detail comes clear in the distance. And that is just the beginning. Limbs that no longer function well, appendages gone numb, turn life's little tasks into an arduous exercise. A gut gone goofy only adds to the chaos.

Strange as it sounds, I do love my life. An imaginative writer could not invent it. My journey wandered off the beaten path long ago. I am a journalist, a recovering network television news producer, who has found more satisfying fare in writing and teaching and doing odd jobs, a day's work for a day's pay.

I am a family man, husband to a lovely and funny woman, a loose cannon named Meredith. Anyone who watches *The View* knows her well. Meredith is the one all the way to the left on your screen. Meredith Vieira is a star rising. But the woman is liable to say just about anything. Life in the home territories is interesting.

I am the father of three gorgeous children with their own view of the world. Ben, Gabe, and Lily are forces to be reckoned with. I reckon they give us gray hair and keep us young. There is a powerful circumstance with which all of us must reckon, however. My health sucks, a condition that has become everybody's problem. Illness is a family affair.

For thirty years, I have done battle with

multiple sclerosis (MS). The disease touches everything I do and affects my body from head to toe. Chronic illness occupies a lowly position in the hierarchy of suffering but takes a toll. By the end of the millennium, I was suddenly clashing with another fierce adversary. Twice in one year, firefights with colon cancer erupted, further compromising the quality of my life.

I have become a magnet for trouble, an aficionado of living on the edge, a most dangerous place for any individual to hang out. The experience has taught me extraordinary lessons about living. Once, I did not know the verb *cope*. Now I know it all too well.

When, fresh out of college, I arrived in Washington, D.C., on a clear spring day more than three decades ago, warm breezes buoyed my feelings of well-being and expectations of a limitless future. Within three years, just as my career as a television journalist was ascending in the historic hurricane of Watergate, I was engulfed in my own, very personal storm. Illness came calling when I was twenty-five years of age, and it has never left.

The once unhampered trek toward a bright horizon has become a shaky walk across moving terrain. The landscape and contours of life have shifted. I have passed from newsrooms through operating rooms to a more reflective existence. The large events of the world, the trembling earth that preoccupies the journalist, have given way to the struggle to sustain a small life.

My thirty-year effort to salvage that life, to wrest it from the clutches of sickness, has been a search for control and the perspective to adjust. Survival skills have been honed, forged in one of life's hottest furnaces. What I have learned is that I am stronger and more resilient than ever I imagined. My dysfunctional vision and impaired body are testaments to the damage MS can inflict. Colon cancer has left me with a gut I could not sell at a used car lot, no money down. But as my body weakens, my spirit grows strong and occasionally soars.

I am not just a collection of muscles and nerves, the wiring that has short-circuited my dreams. Who I am, my very identity rests in my head. It is from that fortress, my command post, that my being takes shape. Citizens of sickness, those who suffer from their own assaults on body and spirit, know disappointment. Ours is a common siege. The battle to control our heads is every bit as important as combating the attacks on our bodies.

The psychological war with illness is fought on two fronts, on the battlefield of the mind and in the depths of the heart. Emotional strength must be learned. I am a better person for that struggle. Attitude is a weapon of choice, endlessly worked. The positive impulse must struggle to survive in a troubled mind. I skirmish with myself, in an effort to shield my eyes from the harsh sight of the diminished person I believe I see looking out from the mirror.

Self-pity is poison. There is no time. I need a future and refuse to become a victim. Too often we become oblivious to our own prisons, taking the bars and high walls for granted. Sometimes we construct them ourselves, and the barbed wire goes up even higher. Too many of the limitations placed on us are an extension of our own timidity.

My weary sighs frequently come with a shrug and the soft statement, "I could write a book." And so, I have. This is my reluctant memoir, a self-conscious stab at an important subject. These pages are not about suffering. That would be tedious. This book is about surviving and flourishing, rising above fear and self-doubt and, of course, anger. Meredith and the children must wear the scars of these epic battles.

And this book is not about sickness but about the search for emotional health. This is not *the* answer, only *an* answer. Coping is a personal art. There is no element of science in coping, no formula or objective standard for measuring proficiency. Coping is measured against only how you want to live and what you think works. I write no prescriptions and do not presume to offer guidance to others. I am just a guy with a fragile grip on my own life, peering through the fog that rolled in during a dream long ago and does not clear away.

I am learning to cope, certainly the toughest course in my continuing education. And the seminar is never over. For me, coping must be relearned every day. Adjusting is not taught at any famous university and will never be advertised on a matchbook cover. Learning to live with adversity is instinctive and self-taught. It is the stuff of life.

So welcome to my world, where I carry around dreams, a few diseases, and the determination to live life my way. This book is my daily conversation with myself. I am happy to share it with you. Life is good. I am happy. My family is intact. My sense of humor flourishes. These pages chronicle the struggles in that exotic place just north of the neck. At the moment, my attitude checks out well. Get back to me tomorrow. I do believe I am winning.

Richard M. Cohen
September 2003

one

A Dream and a Diagnosis

Perhaps I should have seen the ambush coming while I was in college. Warnings came in the darkness of restless nights. There was a foreboding, the uneasy feeling that followed a recurring dream that always unsettled me. Those late-night movies would follow me wherever I traveled and laid my head for the night. They were still playing long after the diploma was in my hand and I had hit the road.

In these dramas, I would be vying fiercely on a basketball court or football field, playing a high-pressure, exquisitely rough game. Always, there was a clock loudly ticking. The action would provide amusement for a while, but as the score got closer and time grew shorter, the pressure became intense. Even in my sleep, I began to sweat.

The contest took on a fierceness that was threatening.

My legs became rubbery. Losing strength, they began to buckle. In the final minutes, with the crowd on its feet and the screaming deafening, I would fall to the floor, ball in hand, no longer able to stand, let alone engage in athletic combat. The team would lose by a single point. The dream was unnerving, and even as it recurred, I did not know what meaning to attach.

More upsetting was the same theme played out in a more threatening, intense arena with my life at stake. This dream was staged on the field of battle, and it came all too frequently. I would be running hard, sweating and breathing wildly. Again, my legs gave out and folded beneath me, leaving me powerless to protect myself from an enemy about to strike a lethal blow. I hyperventilated my way through battle, uncertain that I would survive and always in that fevered state of panic.

Considerable time was spent mulling over these dreams. America was fighting in Vietnam, and I assumed the two dreams reflected my fears of that war. But introspection was not my specialty in the late 1960s and early 1970s. Politics was, and soon journalism would be my calling. I had chosen

Simpson College, a progressive school outside Des Moines, Iowa, as my venue for an education. Simpson was far from home. I needed distance. I was a rebellious middle-class kid from West Hartford, a Connecticut Yankee celebrating the culture of my time and courting all the political conflict a person could handle.

My training as a troublemaker had begun in high school. By graduation, I could have taught the course. I had my early indication that I was temperamentally suited for the future work I would do. In the summer of my junior year in high school, my friends and I broke into the recently abandoned Connecticut State Prison, a medieval fortress at Wethersfield, and stole the ancient electric chair. I thought it was a moment of high meaning. My father saw it as a stupid prank that could not be tolerated. The chair was returned the next day. I have yet to forgive him.

I had been thrown off athletic teams and suspended from school. Getting ejected from class was as routine as eating lunch. Other parents were quietly telling their teenage children to stay away from me. I was such an outcast, a ne'er-do-well on my way to forging a feisty, anti-everything identity, that a career in journalism seemed a logical choice. I certainly did not see myself in the olive uniform that was fast becoming the dress of the day.

The anti–Vietnam War movement consumed me early in college, and I joined the famous "kiddy-crusade," that vast squadron of activists campaigning in 1968 to nominate Senator Eugene McCarthy as the Democratic presidential candidate. Along with my peers, I went "Clean for Gene," my hair respectably cut and beard gone as we sought to dump Lyndon Johnson. I spent the summer in the Southwest and at the riotous Democratic National Convention in Chicago. A lot of us learned at a tender age important lessons about power and politics and the workings of the world that year. I was twenty, and what I took away was the value of perseverance and how to become resourceful, qualities that would rescue me from invisible enemies for the rest of my life. Formative years do write a teaching plan for living. Mine included a toughness that has served me well ever since.

I had been included in the first selective service lottery to determine who would be forced to go to war in Southeast Asia. I watched the dreaded drawing on my ancient black-and-white television. That game of televised roulette was a defining moment for every man in my generation. The lottery was over for me before it ever really started. I trembled as I heard February 14, my birthday, read out and repeated, over and over. It was number 4. That low number guaranteed me a free uniform and at least a one-way ticket to the faraway fight.

I considered going to jail or even to Canada to avoid a war I deeply opposed. Instead I took the easy way out. I escaped the draft and military service with middle-class privilege and a friendly physician's exaggerated diagnosis of a serious neurological condition.

The deception pained me. Presumably, someone drew a higher lottery number and a ticket to terror in Asia instead of me. I did what I thought I had to. I was struggling to survive. We all were, but I was not proud.

I stayed in school and kept working to spread dissent. In 1969, I crossed paths with Peter Jennings, who was then reporting on antiwar activities for ABC radio. I and some of my friends glued ourselves to him for a few days, eating and drinking and talking about politics. Peter had covered the conflict in Vietnam and was willing to talk openly about his life as long as we left the marijuana home. He was passionate about journalism, and I began to rethink my future. That is what I want to do, I thought.

Two years later, I had the new life I wanted. I joined the Washington bureau of ABC News as assistant to the producer of *Issues and Answers*, then that network's Sunday public affairs program. I had made it into the business just in time. Six months later, the Watergate break-in took place and we all learned the names Woodward and Bernstein. After that, news was glorified and every young person in America suddenly wanted to become a journalist. I stuck with ABC for a while, covering Nixon and McGovern and the politics of 1972. These were gripping years. The Nixon presidency was newsworthy, even at its most routine, and the broadcast networks were right in the middle of it. Young people with ambition moved around, however, and the lure of a new place and higher title took me to public television.

I joined a PBS documentary series called *America '73* and was assigned to work on a film about the politics of disability, exploring the life of disabled people and their struggle for government accommodation. Robert "Robin" MacNeil and Jim Lehrer would host the series. My film would mark the beginning of a long collaboration with both men.

On a warm May morning in the nation's capital, I walked down the Hill, passing the Supreme Court and cutting directly through the U.S. Capitol, an easy shortcut in those lazy, low-security days. I wandered into public television's production center, already humming at nine in the morning. I chatted with colleagues and read through transcripts. Then I dropped the coffee pot.

Producers and editors took turns making the coffee. The first to crave a cup just took the initiative to brew the stuff. I was not the first this day, but the pot was empty. The pot was full soon enough, when it slid from my hands, and the hot contents splashed down my leg as the glass shattered against the floor. The accident seemed to occur in slow motion. The mishap felt unusual. The awkwardness of the moment seemed out of place. The container had seemed to just slip from my grasp and tumble away for no apparent reason.

The incident was disconcerting, but I gave it little thought as I continued to work, screening footage and helping to structure the documentary. I was twenty-five years old and healthy, on the fast track as a television journalist. The project was going well, and we were in postproduction, just putting it all together. I had interviewed contemporaries with severe disabilities, some in wheelchairs. One sequence of the film showed me walking around Berkeley, California, with a young fellow in a wheelchair. We discussed the nation's lack of accessibility to public transportation and the many other difficulties that were part of life for the disabled. "Why him and not me?" I had wondered. I thought I would never be able to handle a cane, never mind a chair with giant wheels that I would have to push with my hands to get around.

On this day in Washington, we were sitting at the Steenbeck, an old-fashioned film-editing deck that is seldom seen and little used in today's era of videotape and emerging digital technology. Another portion of the program contained a provocative conversation between Robin MacNeil and a young woman with a severe spinal injury caused by a surfing accident. She, too, sat in a wheelchair and at one point dropped a cup on the floor. I rewound the film a few times and watched the cup leave her hand. Dropping the coffee pot earlier in the day was not lost on me.

At day's end, I walked back up Capitol Hill in blistering heat, heading for my stuffy, third-floor walk-up apartment. We were heading into summer, a brutally hot season in Washington. Already I could see the heat waves shimmering above Independence Avenue. As I stood on a curb facing the Library of Congress, suddenly I lost my balance, then my footing, and had to step into the busy street. It was a small event, except that I was athletic and in reasonably good physical condition. A misstep once more seemed out of character. It just did not feel right.

Walking slowly up East Capitol Street in the heat, I climbed the many steps to the apartment I shared with my wife, Joyce, a childhood friend to whom I had been married for more than a year. Joyce and I already seemed to be moving in different directions, and she was at a rehearsal for a local acting company on this evening. I was alone, not an infrequent configuration with us. My belongings went flying into a corner as I burst into the apartment. I went into the kitchen.

The large old place with its ancient appliances and ripped wallpaper was steamy. I moved to the living room and removed my pants, sitting down on the large old couch to drink a beer. Heat and humidity combined to make the place torturously uncomfortable. A hot breeze blew in through the open window, and I sat as still as possible, dwelling on nothing in particular as I tried to cool off. My left leg itched, and I was idly scratching when I sat up with a start. The outside of the leg was numb. The entire length of my leg seemed almost without feeling on the skin.

Yet another sensation or event that did not feel right was upon me, right smack in my face. The day pieced together like a puzzle, though it formed no discernible shape or design. I did not feel any particular concern, though somewhere inside I began to realize the day's inexplicable events must fit together. I was curious, but reached no conclusion except that another beer was in order. That was frequently my solution to any problems.

Youth was still mine back then, and career concerns always dwarfed anything else. The rest was filed away. The phone rang. It was ABC News, asking if I wanted to work the following month as an associate producer on coverage of Senator Sam Ervin's impending Watergate hearings. My PBS assignment was coming to an end. "Yes," I replied in excitement. "You bet."

These were the days of running to the newsstand in the morning to buy the *Washington Post*. Woodward and Bernstein had to be checked out and *Doonesbury* taken in.

History was being made, and now I would have a piece of it. My adopted world was the nation's capital. Watergate was the best show in town.

The phone rang again. It was my father. We chatted a little, shared our contempt for Nixon, and I casually mentioned the peculiar experiences of the day. The old man listened carefully and asked a few questions, suggesting that I see a doctor, which was overdue anyway. "It cannot hurt," he suggested. "You could stand a physical." We hung up, and I continued sitting, contemplating my new assignment. Minutes later, the phone rang again. The old man had another thought. "I think you have multiple sclerosis," my dad said abruptly.

My father, Benjamin, now eighty-five, is a physician — and he has MS. My dad is an old-fashioned doc, rock-solid and unflappable. The old man usually was cautious in reaching any conclusions. This time he was not. My first coping decision came instantly: Relax and think. I sat back and thought of a day only six years earlier, when I was a college freshman.

I was sitting in a bedroom at our family house with my older brother, Bern, as he tried to explain to my father how it was that he had skied into a tree. I thought it was funny, truth be told, because this smug sibling had been on the slopes that day to teach his stupid brother how to ski. There were chuckles, and then there was silence. "There is something I want to tell you both," my dad said softly.

"I have a disease called multiple sclerosis. Have you heard of it?" he asked. We nodded our heads up and down in silence. I could not even spell the word *sclerosis*. "It can be serious," he went on, "but I probably will not die from it." The old man filled in a few blanks and asked if there were questions. My father's words invited inquiry. His demeanor said otherwise. The announcement had been abrupt, and there was only the sound of the three of us breathing. That brief encounter made little more sense to me than the instant diagnosis I now was hearing through the phone.

The very suggestion of MS entering my life instantly numbed me. The old man's instant diagnosis seemed out of character, if not hysterical, though my twenty-five years of knowing this man told me to pay attention. Usually, he was proved right. This presented a moment of confusion in a life that was otherwise on course. My tolerance for

31

ambiguity was low in general. I did not know enough about multiple sclerosis to realize that a lifetime of ambiguity might lie before me. My doubts were defensive and strong.

Even so, that day of accidents and apprehension was enough to drive me to my internist, who immediately dispatched me to see a neurologist. That doctor quickly made it clear he suspected multiple sclerosis. What else was he going to suspect? My father suffered from MS — and so did his elderly mother, though her diagnosis was never officially pronounced. The diagnostic process was primitive, inefficient, and imprecise in those days.

Little had been said about my grandmother's condition as I was growing up, though it was clear that something had gone wrong with her physically. She had been confined to a wheelchair since my youngest days. There seemed to be an unstated need-to-know standard for sharing personal information in our family. Certainly my father knew that she had MS, but I didn't. I had not known of his illness until I was in college. My radar screen was blank, not even plugged in and turned on. It never occurred to me that I, too, would be in line for a neurological debacle.

Even now I was not convinced I was ill. My minor symptoms had become too big a deal, I thought. Doctors were supposed to be cautious, but they seemed to be rushing to a verdict before the evidence was in. Concern was out of proportion. "No," I calmly explained to my family and friends and doctors. "This is a mistake. I was shooting this PBS documentary about disabled people, and some of them were my age. I liked them. I identified with them. It's psychosomatic. I am really okay." Nobody was buying my explanation, least of all my neurologist. "We will see" was about all he would say. The doctor did use a word that was unfamiliar to me in the context of illness: *denial*.

Fear played no part in my annoyance, or so I assumed. Even though my father had suffered from MS for years, he did not seem to be really suffering. I had not a clue about what living with MS might mean. To me, my dad seemed unscathed by the illness and evidently had done well with his life. "What, me worry?" Alfred E. Newman's sage question became my new mantra. I liked Al. I thought he looked like Ted Koppel.

All roads seemed to be leading to Rome. I was intent on traveling somewhere else. The people in my life seemed too stunned to voice objections. High emotion was visibly absent. Joyce did not seem to react. Perhaps she was confused and kept her upset to herself. My brother, Bern, also my father's son, was unemotional. He, too, was a journalist, working at the Associated Press at the time. My sister, Terrie, was out west and did not know of my possible diagnosis.

My old man, ever the cautious and conservative physician, was hard to read, though he did seem resigned to the diagnosis. Only in my mother, Terry, did I sense a gathering storm. Outwardly, she followed my dad's calm lead, at least in my presence.

My mother was usually calm. She was Earth Mother — all guys my age thought that about their moms — but my longtime friends saw my mom that way, too. Earth Mother was preparing for trembling ground.

The few friends I told of my situation were silent. No one seemed to know anything about MS. Multiple sclerosis certainly sounded serious. So did the heartbreak of psoriasis. There was no perspective in the crowd.

The diagnostic process was slow, and nearly as primitive as in my grandmother's day. There was no nuclear medicine in the early 1970s, no brain imaging. MRIs and CT scans were as much science fiction as the tourist travel into space depicted in the movie *2001: A Space Odyssey*. Neurologists relied on anecdotal evidence and the ultimate weapon, the spinal tap. Grudgingly, I submitted to their inquiries and examinations, but I held off agreeing to the tap until an assignment at work suddenly went haywire.

My boss at ABC News had asked me to go back to the bureau from the Hill, where I was sitting in at the Watergate committee hearings each day, looking on as John Dean implicated President Nixon and H. R. Haldeman and John Ehrlichman hanged themselves. I had to gather and catalogue the videotapes for the library. It should have been an easy-enough task. I simply had to make sure the written logs were included with the tapes and that the tapes themselves were properly labeled and in order. This was grunt work.

I sat alone on the floor in the tape room and quickly became confused. A job that should have taken less than one hour dragged on for many more. I was confounded. Logs and tapes were not matching, and I was putting the wrong documents into the large plastic videotape containers. I began to tremble in anger, choosing combustion over fear. Maybe something really was wrong with me, I admitted to myself for the first time.

I agreed to the spinal tap and checked into the hospital. Curling into the fetal position, I allowed an officious resident to stick a long needle into my spinal column. It did not actually hurt, though the needle's slow entry did produce an electrical tingling sensation. I had to lie flat overnight, the doctor said, or I might get a crushing headache, a condition that a variety of alcoholic beverages were bringing on many nights anyway as I waited to hear my fate.

I knew this final test promised to end the speculation and lay the subject to rest. If the spinal fluid showed clear, so, too, would my future. If the fluid appeared cloudy, the storm would be close behind. How symbolic, I thought. The neurologist would be calling in two days. I had already traveled from denial to recognition of a bad situation and back to believing a giant mistake soon would be exposed.

I was banking on the spinal fluid appearing as clear as a mountain stream, or every fresh, sparkling lake used to brew the bad beer I had grown used to in college. But my emotions were growing thin as the drink and as numb as my leg had been. I could not bring myself to think about the possibility of having MS. The line between lack of sensation and denial is thin. I did not fully understand just what it was I was denying, but it was apparent that I wanted no part of the illness. I had just launched my life.

The appointed hour for my telephone rendezvous with the neurologist came. I was in my apartment alone, planted in a chair next to the door that suddenly took on the appeal of the fire exit. I sat. Waiting. I pulled up the small table with the phone on it. The phone was green, though it should have been hotline red, with a flashing light and siren. I was staring at the phone and jumped when it rang. "You have multiple sclerosis," the neurologist announced coolly. The doctor added a perfunctory "I'm sorry." There was nothing more to say, neither a word of consolation nor a recommendation of treatment.

In those days, it was diagnose and adios. Plan A did not exist. At that moment, my journey to a strange new land began. That place would be both exotic and rude. There would be no certain return. Illness is an unexplored frontier, Virginia Woolf wrote in a 1925 essay. Sickness would take its place with love and war and jealousy as the forces of a newly defined life. They would be joined by coping, a word I did not really know.

There was no treatment for MS. That much I did know from my dad. His symptoms had come on slowly and subtly, which is why his kids were not even aware of the problem until we were out of the house and safely away at school. Now here the words came flying out at me. I heard the official diagnosis, the verdict pronounced by a jury of one. *Ba-da-boom.* Unbelievable. What a mistake this was, and nobody got it, except for me.

There came one quiet emotional reaction late that afternoon. After the phone was returned to the cradle, immediately I wished I could be also. This would be a great time to be an infant again, to be picked up and rocked. I knew that I had heard the truth, but I could not bring myself to believe it. I walked into the bedroom and sat on the edge of the bed, staring out the window at the Capitol, where I had thought my future covering government and politics rested. Now my head was full of visions of hospitals and wheelchairs, and all I could think was, *I am too young for this.*

Then and there, I made the decision not to react. I stared at the Capitol dome. Since I knew so little about MS, there was no response that made sense. There was nothing intelligent I could say or do. There seemed no point in working myself into a frenzy, so I remained quiet. This was my path of least resistance, and I intended to go for a walk. The numbness putting my leg to sleep had spread to my head. I called my father and broke the news to him. "Welcome to the club," he said. "I will pay any out-of-pocket expenses you have," my dad stammered, probably reaching out to me in guilt. "Dad, all your wealth won't buy *me* health," I answered, playing off a Beatles tune.

Thirty years later, I remain at a loss to explain the quiet calm that does not go away. Understated resolve was a knee-jerk response, learned on the spot. My emotions seemed to run a gamut, from A to B. The straitjacket was in place. It came right off the rack, picked out by me. That jacket still fits nicely and stays on my back to this day. The accompanying attitude has guided me through crises on many fronts. The initial decision not to go with the gut, not to flail and freak, may have reflected only the inability or refusal to confront an unpalatable truth.

Serious sickness was a large reality sandwich for a skinny young man to swallow. I seem to have viscerally and quite accidentally stumbled upon a coping mechanism of some value. *Denial.* Misused by amateur shrinks. Misjudged by those who just think it is bad. Misunderstood by those who have not thought it through.

Yes, denial can put the brain to sleep, anesthetizing the mind that refuses to face the truth and see the approaching freight train hauling the heavy load of hard reality. But denial has two sides, and I have been favored by its more attractive side.

For me, denial has been the linchpin of the determination to cope and to hope. Denial allows any individual with a problem to invent his or her personal reality and to move forward with life in the belief that he or she is in control and can do what needs to be done to keep going. Denial encourages anyone to test perceived limits and, as a consequence, to postpone concessions.

There is nothing wrong with that. MS lasts a lifetime, and I have learned that self-knowledge and coping arrive in their own time. I was setting out to prove to the jury of one, me, that I was just like everyone. I was not like everyone anymore, of course, and would not be again, but I could not bring myself to face that simple fact. Not yet.

two

A New Vision

On a chilly morning in October 1973, my eyes flickered open as the sun was rising and horror hit like lightning, lifting me up out of bed, stunned and standing motionless next to the window. I was blind in my right eye. Blind. Totally sightless. The usual early-morning routine of coffee and newspapers in a sunny kitchen was replaced by my own dark headline. I stood, softly mumbling to the empty room, "No. This is not happening."

The videotape in my mind kept replaying. The day before had begun normally. I had been feeling good, living without any of the symptoms of multiple sclerosis I had first experienced since the diagnosis was imposed only four months earlier. But sometime in the morning, a tiny spot, an oil slick on my right eye, just a speck, had suddenly appeared. That spot was a little round puddle that could not be rubbed away, pooling on my window to the world. An afternoon had been spent opening and closing both eyes, hoping to tear up and wash the nuisance away.

Now I was blind. Losing the sight of one eye is a classic manifestation of multiple sclerosis. Even I knew that. As I stood by the bed, wobbling in that chilly bedroom, toes gripping the floor, the terrible truth washed over me. For months I had lived in a house of denial. Now, in one moment, it had given way. It had been a flimsy structure, built on wishful thinking, but it had sheltered me from the heavy weight of a reality I could not bear to confront. Ignorance had been my ally; I had not even asked many questions of the doctors. Silence was an odd tactic for a journalist who, by trade, is all questions all the time. But I did not want to know too many facts. Facts would lead to truth, and truth had been unacceptable. I was facing facts now. I had to admit to myself that I had MS.

Years would pass, however, before I easily and openly acknowledged my illness. Knowledge came slowly, too. I had much to understand about multiple sclerosis, an illness that was then, and even now, little understood. MS is a disease with no sure treatment and no certain outcomes, no cures and no definitive cause. Some experts suspect a virus, others environmental factors. Some think that the human immune system, the body's defense against invading germs and microbes, can be so effective that it occasionally turns on the body itself. And the idea of a genetic component lay far in the future. Finally, I had been drafted, only this time into the army of 350,000 Americans who shadowbox with this neurological enemy they cannot see.

What is evident is that multiple sclerosis is a disease of process, a grim pileup on the highways of the central nervous system. Multiple patches of plaque form where the disease hits motor and sensory nerves after the protective myelin sheath peels away. The illness process is similar to an attack on an old-fashioned telephone switchboard, with its insulation pulling away, short-circuiting phone calls. Signals cross. Life is disrupted. Dreams are derailed.

"Watch out" is what the doctors had been telling me since the diagnosis was pronounced. But because no one could tell me just how my life would change — MS's effects are not uniformly predictable — I had refused to take their warnings seriously.

Now my life was disrupted. Big time.

I entered the hospital reluctantly, my bravado in the dust. The primitive procedures began. Drugs were dispensed with no certain knowledge that they necessarily helped. I endured regular steroid drips, pumped into my arms four times each day. The steroids wreaked havoc on my body, triggering mood swings and, ultimately, depression. "The treatment will kill you if the MS doesn't," a nurse joked.

I gained almost fifty pounds because my appetite and metabolism were thrown off. Some eyesight was restored, a partial remission, but not enough to approach normalcy. Desperation drove me to allow residents to experiment on me, injecting the powerful steroids through my lower eyelid and under the eye itself, a barbaric attempt to reach the damaged optic nerve. I must have been crazy. I visualized the young doctors jumping up and down, squealing in delight, "Oh boy, let's try this now." I was learning to dislike doctors. They treated me as an inanimate object. Through the years, I have elevated that antipathy to an art form.

The next step on the road to reality came with a call from Ted Koppel, my senior colleague at ABC News. Ted had traveled to China with President Nixon on that historic

1972 trip and was in the Asian nation again on assignment. Since a correspondent on the ground in a closed society would likely be the last to know about major events within those borders, we had arranged a system for me to check regularly with a State Department source about Chinese political and military activity. Ted was to call me from China, and I would feed him whatever information I had picked up, disguised, thinly no doubt, as casual conversation.

When Ted's next call from Beijing came, it was rerouted by the ABC switchboard to a number I had given the operators. Our routine conversation about China became an awkward high-volume question-and-answer session about why I was in Georgetown Hospital. "What the hell are you doing there? What is wrong?" Ted asked.

Silence. I did not know what to say. Should I just tell the truth? Nobody at ABC knew anything about my illness or whereabouts. I remember hearing faint, scratchy voices in the distance, jabbering in Chinese, while I was thinking hard about what my response to Ted should be. "I have MS," I finally said softly.

"You have what?" Ted shouted. He must have thought I was referring to MSG, maybe trying to order takeout from him. "Hello? Cohen, I still cannot hear you," he yelled through the phone, knocking me back onto the bed. Phone calls from China were patched though many relay points thirty years ago. "I said I have multiple sclerosis," I yelled back. "Are you deaf?"

The silence grew briefly louder. "I heard you," he said. "Stop shouting." Ted paused. "Take care of yourself." Done. I was out of the closet. With that information, shouted across oceans and continents, crossing political and emotional borders, I finally sealed to myself that I truly did have this serious disease.

Candor had become my first exercise in coping. Open, free-flowing honesty was moving slowly but trickling out, first to myself and then to another. The flow could not be reversed. I knew that. Coping can be a complicated mind game. My life lay before me. I needed some time to figure the new realities out.

My image of self was involuntarily being altered. The person painfully squinting and looking out from the mirror was changing before my eyes. I could see neither this stranger nor the mirror with clarity. I felt powerless, a passenger in a speeding car, the automatic transmission whirring on the steep climb. I was shifting gears, barely aware of the strains of this new uphill adventure.

Change was profound, the loss of control unnerving. Anyone's early years out of school and in the world are all about empowerment. My sense of strength had grown as fast as bamboo. Confidence in the future suddenly was neutralized. The certainty of success had cracked because it was clear now that this illness was going to touch everything that I did from now on. There was no confidence that my vision would return, intact. And it would not. This was going to be a new world for me.

The signs were everywhere. I was unsteady on my feet, bumping into people and furniture, glancing off doorways and tripping on stairs. A lady in the hospital pulled out a cigarette as she sat with guests in the designated visiting area near the elevators (smoking in hospitals was astonishingly common then). I lit a match and went to touch it to her cigarette. I missed by six inches because my lateral perception was so damaged. The lady laughed at me, and I shrank back.

The range of horrors that could become the future was flashing before me. I was staring at the twisted mirrors in the fun house and not having a good time. Damaged goods had replaced the label *winner.* I would be a limited person.

And the beat went on. At one point, doctors thought I might have a brain tumor because of an ambiguous brain scan. Wasn't MS enough? I was fast learning that things always can be worse, an observation that would serve me well in the future. I was strapped down as pressure injections forced dye into my brain in a now abandoned procedure called an arteriogram. A young nurse held my head in her arms. The test was negative, but I was positive my head would explode. The pain and pressure were greater than anything I have experienced in the thirty years since.

Another small epiphany came. Human endurance is of a vast proportion that most of us do not realize. We think we are weak, failing to recognize our intrinsic strength. I was stronger than ever I realized.

In the midst of this chaos in the clinic, Republican lawyers from the Watergate Committee came looking for me, intent on getting information about an ill-conceived campaign espionage plan in George McGovern's 1972 presidential campaign. McGovern's handlers had wanted to steal me away from ABC to spy on Vice President

Agnew. This was before satellites and the era of instant communication, and the McGovern people wanted eyes and ears on the Agnew campaign. The plan had died the death of a bad idea. Now the Republicans were looking for ammunition to fire back at the Democrats.

Events in my life were spinning out of control, even as I was desperately attempting to ground myself in new circumstances. I knew the McGovern thing had been crazy. It would have been an adventure. Composing affidavits now in a hospital room and all the pressure only confused me. Was I being punished for something?

The emotional artillery was out and thundering. I was squirming, finding it difficult to duck while lying in prone position, flat out in a hospital bed. Tethered by tubes, I could not head for any fire exit and run, screaming into the distance. I was stuck with myself. Such thoughts ran through my head in every waking hour, or at least in lucid moments. Much of the time I just lay there, pumped with industrial-strength steroids, additional assorted drugs, and heavy pain medication that dispatched me to La-La Land.

Hey, wait a minute, I bellowed in my head. Stop the show. I'm only twenty-five. I don't need this. I'm out of here. Not so fast, reality answered.

When I finally left the hospital, I was still shaking. And I was angry. Anger was new, first noticed when my passion for tennis had turned to frustration a season earlier, before I had been told I had MS. I could no longer hit the ball well. My temper flared. After the diagnosis, I quit the game.

I regretted losing tennis and later told my friends that multiple sclerosis had been visited upon me only because I had acted like such a baby, throwing my tennis racquet over the net and otherwise exhibiting juvenile competitive behavior on the court. I had played so aggressively, in pursuit of conventional success. That was how I wanted to live. The zen of the game had been misplaced, though, which became an apt metaphor for the life that would follow.

Anger would become the new companion on my journey, hanging close and never straying too far. My anger on leaving the hospital was explosive. I erupted at anything that moved, autos that cut me off and people who crossed my path. One day I drove a friend to Union Station. My right eye was still functionally gone; I was struggling to see beyond the vague blur. The auto was freedom to me, and the possibility of its loss had me desperate with fear.

Tossing my friend's parting gift into the trunk, I bent down, simultaneously noticing three wine glasses in an open box and bashing my head against the corner of the open trunk door. The wine glasses instantly disintegrated, becoming a thousand glass shards spread throughout the trunk. My bellowing turned heads. Six months of uncertainty growing into acknowledgment of serious sickness had ignited spontaneously.

I had wanted to be larger than life. The fantasy was over. I no longer saw myself as the swashbuckler, starring as the Errol Flynn character in the movie of my life. The trouble with men is that we cannot forget that once we were boys. And boys see their lives as cinema until we are forced to grow up, to walk away from the theaters in our heads and go home to reality.

But what was my reality to be? I made a halfhearted round of visits to some experts, seeking advice as to what I could do. They offered platitudes and slightly forced hope for the future. When doctors focus their hopes on the future, confidence in the present cannot ride high. I decided that any sentence beginning with the word *someday* was not worth finishing.

Then my neurologist recommended a thin volume by a former director of St. Joseph's Hospital in Tacoma, Washington, which specialized in the treatment of multiple sclerosis. The MS clinic there closed in 1959. I had no trouble figuring out why. Published in 1962, *Living at Your Best with Multiple Sclerosis* opened with "A Creed for Those Who Have Suffered." "I asked God for strength," an ode to attitude began, "that I might learn humbly to obey." MS was being presented as an emotional tithe. Very useful.

This small book went on to offer three simple steps for dealing with the onset of serious problems stemming from multiple sclerosis. The first chapter recommended that sufferers "apply three simple emotional 'first aid' measures: (1) take several deep breaths; (2) don't talk for a time; (3) *keep smiling*" (their italics). Excuse me? Who is smiling?

When I finished my dark snickering, a more sobering thought crept into my consciousness. Attitude is not to be so easily dismissed as a source of power and influence governing the course of a disease. Smelling the flowers and thinking good thoughts would not deliver health, I was reasonably sure. Staying strong and maintaining a positive outlook might. Here was my small raft in a choppy sea, difficult to cling to, yet all that I had. Intuitively, I knew that my psychological well-being would be as important to my health as any detours my body would take.

Denial of the diagnosis was evolving into a refusal to accept limitations and the determination to keep my life on track. Learning to survive and to adapt to new and threatening circumstances was my mission now. My course became simple, if not functionally simplistic. Admit illness. Control emotion. Limit knowledge. Preserve the prerogative to deny, to pad the present and make the most of a compromised life. This maneuvering was a variation on the old head-in-sand two-step. I was keeping my head down but trying to look straight ahead, albeit through a cracked lens.

The year 1973 became a preface to the next thirty years. I learned my first lessons about coping and coexisting with a threatening illness. Presuming control when such does not exist was folly. Failing to see the truth had slowed me down. Those fictions only made the climb steeper. I did not know what to think of myself anymore because serious sickness somehow felt like it was my fault. I was being punished. That was a childlike response, but there it was.

I had a new view of myself as diminished, and it hurt deeply. I felt cheated and defeated, and I was in sore need of resurrection. The process of rising up could begin only from within. For me, adapting to illness seemed quiet and personal, appropriately, a solitary pursuit. But if I looked outside myself, I could see two stalwart souls who also struggled with the neurological nightmare: my grandmother and my father. I did not think of them consciously as role models, but they were.

three

Family Legacies

There is an old saying in the news business: Go with what you've got. Deadlines do not wait for perfection. In 1974, there was no perfect solution in sight for me, only my own deadline for moving forward. Time had passed. Ground had been lost. My dreadful year was over, my world calmed. I now faced a life with multiple sclerosis, and I was confused, struggling to adjust to a new reality. My eyes fixed on those who had taught me the essential rules of engagement with illness: my grandmother Celia and her elder son, Benjamin, my father. In a sense, I went home.

Celia Shedroff Cohen was unusual for her time. She owned and operated the Patricia Ladies Shop on Albany Street in Schenectady, dating back to the late 1930s. Tough and independent, she was one of the first women in the state of New York to drive an automobile. That was part of the family lore of my youth.

Grandma Cohen had her own way of doing just about everything. She gave up a bad cigarette habit, a pack a day of Camels, and an unsatisfactory domestic arrangement, marriage, in her adult years. She did not care what others thought; she knew what she needed in her life.

The woman elevated eccentricity to an art form. A doting mother to her two sons, she believed that Benjamin became a physician because she sat in a cemetery reading medical textbooks while she was pregnant with him. This paternal grandmother loved to joke with her grandchildren, to throw back her head and say with a signature laugh that she might as well live it up because she would never live it down. Celia referred to my cousins, her other grandchildren, as "the girl" and "the boy," though she knew them from birth. She was a bit strange, but her spirit never suffered.

Celia was strength personified, even as she slowly lost her ability to walk. Celia never sought medical help without prodding nor actually was diagnosed with MS. By the time her doctors realized that this neurological illness was what had put her in a wheelchair and, ultimately, into a nursing home, the lady was elderly, and no doctors wanted to put her through the ordeal of an imprecise, often lengthy diagnostic process. The doctors finally knew that she had been stricken with MS, though I doubt she ever did.

Celia died when I was thirty-two. I got the call one cold winter day and headed for the train to Hartford, where she had finished her life. I remember thinking on that trip to Connecticut that Celia never had seemed to be held hostage to her illness, though, of course, she was. Somehow, she rose above it. I never heard her complain about her health. She took each day at a time. She had more on her mind than herself. Celia liked people well enough. She loved animals. Once, when I visited, she noticed ants on the floor and would not move her wheelchair for fear of crushing them.

Celia's determination not to complain and never to hurt any creature kept her going. Though we have told stories about her in the family and shared a lot of laughs, her eccentricity could not obscure the lessons of how to live gracefully.

My grandmother seemed to accept and live with her limitations. Grandma never knew what she was dealing with. The initials

MS probably meant nothing to her. Perhaps ignorance brought peace. I ask myself if I want to or even could adjust that peacefully. I of course live with a declared diagnosis which has reshaped my view of the world. And, too, I am always ready for the fight. I struggle with doubt about the virtue of accepting one's burdens without a struggle.

Then again, when is a fight smart? Celia showed no anger, revealed no bitterness about her life. This grandmother began to define what would become the bedrock tenets of our family culture, a strong value system that told her to adapt and to keep going. My father learned the lessons she taught well.

The daily histology class at Albany Medical College in 1938 brought first-year medical students to the microscope with frequency. The course was a requirement. Decembers in upstate New York could turn bleak, but life seemed sunny for my future dad, then only twenty. College was over, a new life begun. The late autumn brought with it the numbing routine of the long haul just under way. One particular day would present a life-changing surprise. Peering into a microscope, one eye at a time, slowly and methodically, brought the startling realization to this aspiring doctor that he was completely blind in one eye.

"I saw absolutely nothing," the old man remembers. "I had used the same eye on the same scope the day before without a problem. It took a microscope to show me I had the problem because the other eye was functioning normally, and looking at a distance, I could not appreciate what was happening." Your brain was compensating, I suggested. "Those are your words," my dad quickly replied, ever dispassionate and clinical. A third quality came into play during this first crisis in what would become a long ordeal. Calmness.

My dad did not know what had gone wrong in his body. Neither did the medical school professors who suddenly became his doctors. They thought the loss of sight was psychogenic, a medical term for "all in his head." The advice he got was to quit medical school, because it was apparent he could not handle the pressure. He went home, and miraculously, the sight returned. It would take years for him to know that sight loss in one eye is not uncommon in multiple sclerosis, and neither is a full or partial remission.

Double vision set in toward the end of medical school, but again he got scant feedback and no wisdom from the doctors he saw in the wards and on the floors so regularly. "When World War Two finally broke out, like all of my classmates, I went for a physical examination to be taken into the armed forces," my dad says today. "By chance, I was examined by a young neurologist who told me that without question, I had a systemic neurological condition. That was as precise as it got." Turned down by the navy, he stayed in school.

"How disappointed were you?" I ask. His contemporaries were leaving their lives, whatever their calling, donning uniforms to fight America's enemies in Europe and the Pacific. "It was a blow," the old man says. "I went to that exam without any medical history and could not get in. Something was wrong."

This was the beginning of the war boom. For the young people, mostly men, who had grown up and managed to get through school, then more school, during the Depression, success generally came at a high price. The determination to succeed and the hard work it took to make dreams happen forced young people to focus and grow up fast.

My dad did just that. He knew what he wanted and went after it. Life, after all, is a meritocracy. Happiness is earned, at least until serendipity steps in with that inevitable moment that proves the silly assumption untrue. The hard lesson that life is not fair came early to my dad, though he could not have known that this was just the beginning.

My father simply went about his business. As his physical problems increased across the years and into my adulthood — he became unsteady on sidewalks and stairs, even falling from time to time, though we children were never told — so, too, did his determination to live his life as he, not some other doctor, saw fit.

"When limitations came on, I just went along with them," he remembers, almost casually. "I did not involve myself with histrionics, saying, 'Oh lord, I am going to be a cripple.' I just went day to day." That is the crux of the coping challenge, to keep the ball in play and the door to dramatics shut tight. "I am not sure of the future," he says, "but I will take it as it comes." Adjust, after the fact. Do not simply react to possibility.

This seems so elementary, except that people seem to have great difficulty holding on to perspective. More often than not, I am convinced, this is less the function of a conscious choice than internal makeup and emotional carriage. "People do not consciously decide. It is more subconscious, a matter of personality and how they are put together," the old man adds.

Coping has been a quiet quest for my dad, even within the family and across generational lines. Nobody talked much about multiple sclerosis. Celia kept her counsel. "If she had physical problems, she never would have told her children," my dad reports. And did the old man tell his mother about his MS? "Well, I never told my parents anything," my father reports. "I think they would have died to know I had a problem." His brother, Aaron, now eighty-two, a retired executive with the Economic Development Administration in the U.S. Department of Commerce, told me, "Your father does not like to deliver bad news. He would rather keep it to himself."

In his actions and attitude, his behavior inside and outside the family, my father seemed to believe in discretion bordering on silence. He had not often discussed the illness with anybody, even with my mother, his wife of fifty-eight years. "Of course I knew that something might be wrong," my mom remembers. "We were way past questions of medical school hysteria by the time we married," she says, pausing thoughtfully. "Multiple sclerosis was a possibility," she says, "not a probability."

By the time the pieces started to fit together in his mind, the pattern of keeping to himself was well established in the old man's playbook. "When he had a problem, he solved it, and then he told me," my octogenarian mom says to me matter-of-factly. Theirs was a marriage of a different time, when men were men and everyone else was kept in the dark.

Patriarchal prerogatives stood my father alone at the helm. And it seems old-fashioned male behavior to simply suffer in silence. No one in our house doubted my father's love. Family and medicine were his life. With unqualified devotion, he embraced both. The old man is of a different time, and he operated in a very different social context. And he is weird.

"There were two reasons," my mother says, explaining my dad's attitude. "One being, well, that's the way he has always been. The other, he was afraid that information could hurt his career. He had patients' lives in his hands. They might have said, 'I cannot take a chance.'" That is a very old story.

"Physician, heal thyself," Aesop wrote as the moral to an ancient fable. The sick, it was believed, should not treat the sick. Only the healthy can close wounds. My dad's concern seemed to be valid enough in a world of prejudice and ignorance about illness. Those suffering from serious illnesses certainly hid in closets across America for many years. Why should this family be any different?

When my diagnosis came, barely thirty years after my father's graduation from medical school, the old man skipped the health implications and went right to the heart of the challenge: controlling the information. "Do not tell anyone," he quickly advised. "This information can be used against you." For once, I did what I was told.

The old man's fear for me was a logical extension of his experience, if not the wisdom of the time. Loose lips sink ships. A journalist and television news producer surveying the lives of others could be compromised by public knowledge of this strange and threatening disease. This was a matter of self-defense. I was too new to the adult world to dispute his logic.

Eventually, I would chart a different course. The choices I made mixed a more enlightened, if naïve, consciousness with realistic common sense. An instinct to survive and the need for self-protection are strong. Eventually, the curtains did come open.

The light was bright. The heat felt warm. At the same time, I learned to protect my back in dealing with others. In the end, we all are at the mercy of other people, and I would learn the hard way that trust must come slowly and selectively.

four

Candor Conundrum

Late morning usually brought the day's first fast break from school, the hazardous dash through traffic and across Broadway, a jay-running junket for coffee and whatever offered a sugar fix to graduate students facing another long day. My poison of choice was Reese's Peanut Butter Cups. The hypersweet, cloying candies had become jet fuel for my flight through Columbia University's journalism school. I was attending Columbia to hone my writing and production skills. Also, I did not have a job.

I had kicked around ABC News doing documentary work after returning to active duty from those forced idle days and weeks in the hospital. The 1973 oil embargo had dried up the economy, and the shock waves were still registering a few years later. Cutbacks at the networks came, and I went. Unemployed and unhealthy, I was unhappy as I headed back to school, uncertain that the move had been right. Sight in my right eye was running at half speed as I hurtled full speed, determined to get through Columbia and jump-start my flagging career.

I was already wired as I was launched on my Broadway sugar binge in the late winter of 1976. The end of the school year was in sight and my master's degree within reach. I wanted badly to be done and gone, heading back to work in the real world. I was not feeling quite right that morning but could not put my finger on what the problem was.

The sunlight was blinding as I stood on Broadway, peering uncomfortably into the distance and waiting to cross as buses and cars came speeding down the wide avenue.

Traffic slowed, then stopped. I looked up and across the road, ready to walk, trying to blink away the glare and search for the pulsating green sign instructing me to walk. The marker was nowhere to be seen. But it had to be there. I peered hard, frantically straining to scan the other side of Broadway for that identifiable green command or, for that matter, any recognizable landmark in the hodgepodge of businesses at 116th

Street by Columbia's main quadrangle. There was only the blur of outlines and movement. Finally it dawned on me that something was very wrong.

My good eye was going. Since my right eye had dimmed in 1973, I had depended on other senses and my left eye to survive the perils of pedestrian life in the big city. Now my other eye was going dark. Ears immediately picked up where eyes left off. The compensation of one sense for another was instantly apparent as I dodged back across Broadway, just trying to keep my balance.

I hurried back into the school and spent the afternoon testing my vision. I discovered I could not read words of any size print in any book, magazine, or newspaper under any conditions. A trip to Columbia's medical center the next day introduced me to a first-rate neuro-ophthalmologist, a straight shooter. "On any given day," he warned, "for the rest of your life, there will be a fifty-fifty chance that you will lose more eyesight."

My parents descended from Connecticut. My mother was devastated, bursting into tears in a restaurant as she watched me press a menu against my face, still unable to read it. I was unnerved. Displays of high emotion were unusual in the family culture.

Others at the table, my brother and his girl-friend, just stared straight ahead at nothing.

My father broke the ice, advising all to stay calm. "Something will happen. Things will change, one way or another," the old man said. "That's how this disease works." I was back in the business of learning about MS.

Once again, I was numb, feeling almost nothing. A circuit breaker seemed to have kicked in. There was not even a sense that I had been screwed. Screw that, I thought. My eyes had to face forward, even if they did not see so well. I vowed that I would not be affected by this problem. That, of course, was absurd. I was deeply affected already. My vision was approaching legal blindness just as the end of school had come into sight.

My failing vision presented me a world of illusions. Reality bent. I was trying to sort out what I saw and make sense of what I thought I saw. They were not always the same. Objects changed shape and size according to light and distance. A German shepherd sprawled on the floor across a room might become a footlocker as I walked closer.

The surprises seemed never to end. I was sitting on the step down into a friend's living room one evening. Sudden movement registered in my peripheral world, the clearer field of vision off to the side. My head jerked to the right, quickly scanning the room to spot the intruder. The space was empty. Then I saw. Slipping to my knees, I bent over an ant moving across the room. That I could spot that little guy out of the corner of my eye stabbed me with the reality of what I could not see directly before me. I was quickly realizing I no longer lived in the land I once knew.

What I could no longer see was unambiguous, though. I saw and literally felt the visual barriers surrounding me, closing me in. Sometimes I felt intensely claustrophobic, as if walls were moving in. I still experience those sensations.

The vagaries of images around me — strange shapes in the distance, vehicles flashing by, or people suddenly appearing out of the fog — were everywhere. My wrecked vision was disorienting. I longed to break through that barrier. This was all new to me. Details disappeared quickly as I sat back, staring out any window and into the distance. Even movies were no longer an option. The silver screen, as with all of life at any distance, had become an impressionist painting, objects fading into shapeless blurs. The painting has remained on that easel.

And my career took on the feel of memory. My world had centered on a visual medium. I was a television news producer, going down, I thought, for the third time. I could not see, never mind sort out, the images on a television monitor. Sorting out life and the world was what journalism was supposed to be all about. Even finishing graduate school was thrown into doubt. My old life had passed away.

To say I was freaked does no justice to the concept. I knew I had to tell someone at Columbia what was happening, even if that was at war with the Cohen family obsession of secrecy and silence. But whom to trust was the difficult question.

Fred W. Friendly, who led a seminar on media and society, drew the short straw. The volatile and bombastic former president of CBS News and, before that, producer and partner of Edward R. Murrow, scared me to death. Fred accepted no excuses for the job not done. "Don't tell me your troubles," he would snarl to any student looking for the easy way out. Easy was not on my wish list. A way out of this mess was. I didn't expect compassion from Fred either, but that wasn't my priority; no amount of coddling was going to help me recover my sight. Fred was a no-nonsense guy, and I was in need of unvarnished guidance from someone with good instincts and strong survival skills. I took a deep breath and paid Fred a visit.

Ever the consummate journalist, Professor Friendly responded to my account of my progressive illness by insisting that he needed to speak privately to my neurologist and hear the story directly from him. Fred would not even take the phone number from me. He wanted to track down the doctor himself to make sure there were no tricks on my part. The man took nothing for granted.

When Fred reached the neurologist and was satisfied that in fact my situation was real, he began to teach me more than journalism. Fred showed me first that he cared, something few doctors had ever bothered to do. Fred made it clear that he was upset and had his own coping to do. I was surprised but instantly comforted.

Fred's instinct in that moment was gentle. He knew that I was wounded and vulnerable, and he sensed I needed something more than advice about how to make it through the rest of the academic year and get that master's degree. That became the easy part. I sat through long sessions in his office as he proceeded to talk about his former wife's grueling psychological problems. Fred spoke in highly personal terms about her institutionalization and the impact that had on his family.

Fred did not have to do that. He was baring his soul for a reason. In sharing the stories of his emotionally painful ordeals and how he learned to grapple with them, he was offering his life as metaphor for mine. Fred was telling me I was not alone. He was also teaching me that it is safe to tell others about a bad situation.

"Be honest," Fred advised. "Be open. Talk." Tell prospective employers the complete truth about your medical problems, he counseled. That is the honorable thing to do. "They are going to find out anyway," he said. "Better coming from you." Fred also warned me I would have to be a better producer than any and all competitors for jobs in television news, to compensate for my limitations.

"I have seen your work," Fred added, leaning forward in his chair. "Frankly, you are not that good," he said in his matter-of-fact way. That vote of no confidence may have been well intentioned, but it hurt. For me, there was no turning back now. I had not come this far and climbed these hills to suddenly choose a new career. I had a strong take on Fred's advice to me. I believed that in the end, Fred was trying to protect me from an unkind marketplace, to steer me away from certain disappointment. Fred stood by his call for honesty. Decades later, I believe he felt that candor was the proper approach and I would be eaten alive.

Fred had a longstanding tradition of introducing his best and brightest graduate students at Columbia to CBS News and lobbying for jobs for them. The list of recipients of his successes was long. He made no such overtures on my behalf. That did not surprise me. I knew Fred thought I should pack it in and leave the business. He knew that news executives had little patience for the problems of employees. Lord knows he hadn't when he was running the show at CBS. But my credo in dealing with illness had become "Never give up." Fred was protecting me. To hell with Fred Friendly, I thought. I was moving forward.

As graduate school was ending, I had a job interview at *NBC Nightly News*, where the executive producer early in the year had expressed interest in meeting with me after Columbia, almost promising me a job. I came ready to speak the truth.

The *Nightly* newsroom was situated on the fourth floor at Rockefeller Center, overlooking the skating rink where the tree stands every Christmas. The executive producer told me there were jobs in Washington and Los Angeles, and that he would seriously consider me for either. Then I told him about my illness. At first he said nothing. He sat up straight, tugging on the knot of his necktie. His back stiffened. I thought I heard the click as the light in his eyes went out. "There is a lot to think about," he said. "I will get back to you." He never did.

I learned a valuable lesson then and there. Honesty is not the best policy. Candor about health problems works in the confines of academia and maybe in the movies. Full disclosure does not work so well in the real world. Hard times in a competitive industry at a tough moment in history leave little room for dealing fairly with a serious illness. People with serious problems can be perceived as weak candidates for employment in the dollars-and-cents world. The right thing to do has currency when nothing is at stake. News may be a calling that honors truth, but that truth sets no one free.

Don't tell nobody nuthin'. My old man

was right. Truth had some appeal, but I outgrew it; obfuscation was where I was headed. The moral imperative to bring honesty to the table turned in my mind to a strategy of the passive lie. I went back to public television, to *The MacNeil/Lehrer Report*.

The decision not to talk about MS, to keep the disease under wraps, was an act of self-defense. But it did not come without cost. Silence undercut my ability to adjust to the disease. I was hiding something, and secrecy felt dirty, as though I had done something wrong. The recesses of the mind are dark. The information hiding there only grew darker, too. I have never lost that feeling of culpability.

My stealth approach bothered me enough to write my private rulebook outlining when dishonesty went too far and when it was permissible. In the marketplace, where all of us are hostages, I would take no chances. Never take an open mind for granted. In my personal life, though, candor was a requisite, but in varying degrees.

"Cohen, why can't you see better?" "What's wrong with your sight?" "You seem blind as a bat." Budding journalists have such a way with words. If one Columbia classmate posed that idle question, it seemed as if they all did. My stock answer sufficed. "Bad eyes." That was it. Bad eyes. "Oh, okay," the interrogators invariably replied, revealing the lack of real concern that prompted me to wonder why the questions were posed in the first place.

If people wanted to know, invariably they would find their way to the fountain of truth anyway. Many of my close friends were in the news business, and everyone knows that journalists cannot keep secrets. I leaked the information to a select group. My theory is that if a secret is juicy enough, a person learning the sexy truth will have to tell one person. Just one. You cannot resist it. That individual, of course, will have to inform yet another. By that calculus, the city knows what is happening soon enough.

Truth would be pushed in faces impulsively, even prematurely, in the not-too-distant future. A chip was growing, riding high on my shoulder. Deep in my head, I silently dared others in my life to walk away. Joyce was already fleeing to a different place in her life. This was not an easy situation.

Others learned the truth in mysterious ways. When I went against the old man's wishes and told my childhood pal Andy, he soon reported back that his mother already knew the truth about my health. Another lesson: There are no secrets in a community that cares. We only pretend we own exclusive rights to the truths of our lives so we can assure ourselves we are in control of our fates.

PBS was televising the debates between Gerald Ford and Jimmy Carter in the 1976 presidential election. I was in Philadelphia, the site of the first face-off, interviewing voters and screening possible panelists to watch the debates with MacNeil and Lehrer and evaluate the event. I approached a middle-aged woman walking through Center City in the heart of the historic downtown district.

This pleasant lady was intelligent and opinionated, the perfect television guest. I decided on the spot to invite her to join us. "How long would this take?" she asked.

"Oh, this will go all evening," I answered, "at least three or four hours." The woman seemed to freeze, then stepped back. "No," she said quietly. I just looked at her. "My husband has multiple sclerosis," she told me. "I could never leave him alone for that long." I seemed to freeze, too, squinting and trying to see her face more clearly, searching for sense in that moment.

The open honesty seemed stunning. A

lady I did not know was telling me a painful truth, an intimate fact passed along to an imperfect stranger. How odd, I thought. Why would she do that? I pondered the risk of such openness. Clearly, there was none. She offered information as if truth-telling was second nature rather than unnatural.

That observation came as an epiphany. I had never met anyone outside my family who lived with MS, never mind talked about it. The woman told me that she and her husband had traveled the world seeking a cure for multiple sclerosis. I hope MS never owns me and I never do that, I thought. Her candor was not lost on me, however, and I knew I had a lot to learn. My stare must have been intense, because the conversation was over but the woman gazed at me in silence and did not move.

I felt an urge to share my secret story, to embrace her and assure her that I understood. My mouth opened, but no words sprang forth. My uncomfortable silence puzzled me. I felt bad that I was not reaching out to this person. A gesture on a busy street corner would have been generous. I smiled weakly through my locked jaw. That was all I could do.

My secret was safe.

But I was in transition, the candor issue only a piece of the puzzle still spread on the table. The larger quest was for control and confidence. My power had been compromised, and I needed to feel strong again. My eyes had become my most difficult problem and the most potent symbol of the weakness in my life.

A powerful dream had played at the theater of my head in the turbulent months after that loss of vision. To this day, the film or variations rerun with some frequency. In the drama I am driving, tooling along on an old and winding highway up the Hudson. I am hyperaware of colors, the blue sky, the green trees, the bright flowers, all of which, in reality, have gone pale in my eyes.

As I drive, a fog rolls in, quickly growing thicker and more billowy. Soon I can no longer see the road ahead. I choose the accelerator over the brake, speeding to the point of danger. Believing that I will drive through the fog that is blinding me, I increase my speed until, uneventfully, the dream comes to a close.

In my head and in my hopes, I had it that I would see clearly again. That was not to happen. Power in my life would need to be regained in other ways and the issue of eyesight laid to rest. The hope of bringing honesty and success into my life, together and in tandem, yin and yang, seemed only a fantasy. Candor and career were rivals, if not enemies, and I predicted a long war.

five

Racing Against MS

Hard news was where the action was, the place most every young television journalist wanted to be. The evening news was the arena I had yet to enter. Troubled health and limited eyesight kept my expectations low, thrusting the romantic world of the evening news into the distance. The Cronkite crowd I grew up watching would probably remain as distant figures on the tube.

My sphere had centered on documentaries and live television. With no formula known to me for making the right connections and breaking into daily news, I was fast becoming a creature of PBS. In the spring of 1979, I sat in my office at WNET, New York public television, reading a news item in *Variety*.

The short article announced that CBS

News had appointed a Director of Recruitment, a job title I associated more with a football team than with the television news business at that time. Impetuously, I stuck a piece of stationery into the typewriter and wrote this stranger a note. I announced to him, all too glibly, "I do not know what you are recruiting for, but if it is not the army, sign me up." The overture was foolish. I heard nothing back and felt mildly embarrassed.

Summer had arrived, and I gave CBS News little thought. When this mysterious man did contact me, I was shocked to hear from him. He was gruff and promised nothing. He growled and told me he had checked me out, then dispatched me to meet various broadcast producers and, finally, the guys in the white shirts of the front office.

"Don't embarrass me," my new patron snarled. "You are my first candidate."

I made the rounds at CBS; no one asked a single personal question, and I offered no personal information. By summer's end, I was offered a producing job on the *CBS Evening News with Walter Cronkite*. When the call came, I was thrilled for an opportunity I once considered out of reach. There was a contract to negotiate, some routine paperwork to sign, and, oh yes, the company physical to take at CBS corporate headquarters in New York, a black-stone-sheathed building informally known as Blackrock.

A physical? This was a bolt out of the blue. Instantly I realized that once again I would face difficult choices about truth and health and the self-protection of silence. My predicament played into the siege mentality that comes too easily with illness. The world was not against me. It just felt that way. I was torn between a winning strategy and a losing brush with conscience. I called my friend Robert MacNeil. "Robin, I do not know what to do," I lamented, if not whined. "Do you think I should tell them everything?"

A pause followed. "No, I do not. Say nothing," MacNeil advised. "Your silence," he said, "is an honorable dishonesty." At last, a person I respected mightily had given me permission to lie. The words *health* and *honor* begin with the letter *h*. The *h* is silent in *honor*. (Years later, Sanford Socolow, Cronkite's executive producer, told me that I had done the right thing. "I am not proud to say this," he said quietly, "but I don't think I would have hired you if I had known.")

I felt dirty, but not too dirty. So much of what I had learned about journalism had to do with basic honesty and full disclosure. Yet there I was, about to perform a dishonest act to inaugurate my relationship with an institution built around honesty. This was a fine kettle of fish.

All that stood between the Cronkite newsroom and me now was the company physical. Such exams are not known for their attention to detail, and I figured I probably could bluff my way through the ordeal. It was the eye examination that worried me most, but I had a plan. My right eye was considerably more damaged than the left — some vision had eventually returned in my left eye — so I would test the left eye twice. How, I did not know. I took the exam, patch over my right eye first. "Now cover your left eye," the nurse instructed. "I just did," I answered sweetly. "My mistake," she responded, with a smile. "Then cover your right eye." I was happy to oblige.

I passed the physical.

The push to get to CBS had been so consuming that I had given little thought to how I would pull off the responsibilities and many physical challenges if I succeeded. All I had to do now was be brilliant in a new job, in an area, daily news, where I had no experience. And I had to be better than any seasoned, healthy producer on the job. That is what I believed. When my new masters at CBS News learned the truth about me, and they would, I feared I would be held to a different standard from that applied to my colleagues. I had dissembled to get the prized position. My bosses could not like that. And this society honors, indeed celebrates, physical perfection, turning away from the sight of the afflicted. I was jumpy, already covering my ass in my head. The pressure on me was self-generated and intense.

The celebrations were few and short-lived. There was work to be done. My time would be theirs. There were no conflicts with the rest of my life.

My five-year marriage to the girl from my youth had ended peacefully a few years earlier. That was no headline. Differences in expectations and the facts of our lives sent us into separate orbits. I knew I wanted children. Joyce said she did not. This was not to be. Scars were few. No runs. No hits, I figured. One error, and two left out in the cold.

CBS News was nerve-wracking and, at the same time, great. I was working closely with many of the correspondents I had watched on television after dinner as I was growing up. Cronkite and Collingwood, Moyers and Mudd were my heroes. Work was exhilarating, and nobody knew my secret. I began to doubt that the secret existed, always quick to deny, deny, deny.

I was a producer on the *CBS Evening News with Walter Cronkite*, and my position had empowered me to forget the rest. My bosses did not send me out on stories for a while, choosing instead to keep me around the news desk and tape room to learn the ropes. The evening news producers were a close-knit group. Colleagues explained to me that they usually hit the ground first on a story, renting a car and scoping out the situation before the camera crew or correspondent arrived. Renting a car would be a problem, driving it a disaster. I did not even possess a driver's license and had not in years. I knew that sooner or later, this would mean trouble. Planning logistics was my quiet nightmare. I was constantly immersed in planning ahead, always in a panic.

In my mind, my life at CBS News pitted me against everyone else. They walked with such swagger and seemed to do their jobs so effortlessly that I felt threatened, which was odd, because I liked my colleagues so much. They were my new friends. They were my enemies. They could not know.

I finally told the truth to my boss. That event came when I felt secure and was sick of the cover-up. I realized I could little afford for the truth to come from a source other than me. Reaction was strong. There was shock, then muted discomfort on executive row and a self-conscious confusion about what to say and do. The front office, of course, knew nothing about the illness or what it would mean, so ignoring my news seemed to be the appropriate course of inaction.

Later I learned that the subject had been discussed in the front office in terms of company liability. My fear was that my boss might now see me as a liability. But the great issue faded into the blur and white noise of the newsroom. Most of my colleagues and contemporaries heard nothing. "Now, why did you have to tell us" was the unspoken response. My duty finally had been discharged.

But while I no longer feared the truth, I should have feared the substance of that truth. My illness was a ticking bomb inside of me. I had been too preoccupied with hiding its existence to dwell on its possible consequences. I was already close to legally blind, a distinction that would come soon enough. And though my health was okay otherwise, I knew that multiple sclerosis does not stand still for long. Common sense advised me that my health and fortunes would turn sooner or later.

Not now, though. There seemed to be time. I continued to sprint, assuring myself that I was outrunning the disease. My dues had been paid in those first couple of years on the evening news. Grunt work was my specialty. I covered economic news, the equivalent of time in the pit. I cut pictures for other people's stories, mastering the technical skills I needed as I went. I covered the fires and floods, explosions and assorted disasters, the picture stories that are the meat and potatoes of television news.

And then Dan Rather became anchor, and my life changed. I had become Dan's producer and friend. Opportunities began to present themselves and I was ready. I soared to the apogee of my denial. Dan had assumed the throne with enormous power, and I was a confidant. That status was validation for me, not so much for the power it implied but for the value I believed others saw in my work. My sense of myself as invulnerable for now was not challenged by the slow progression of the MS. My wings were spread wide.

My first overseas assignment gave me the

chance to cover a major breaking story. Poland and the emerging trade union movement known as Solidarity were on front pages around the globe, and the world was watching. This would mean going into a Communist country at war with itself. Journalists were followed and harassed in Warsaw. I still could not see across the street and was beginning to feel increasing weakness on my right side. I was in the throes of my new counterphobia, the need to do whatever scared me the most.

The visa arrived. I grabbed my passport, condescendingly bought chocolate and nylons for the natives, and left for Poland. My assignment served many agendas. My job had taken on new meaning. Working with the best was not only a privilege, it also made me feel whole, just like them. No illness known to humanity was going to stop me.

The overnight flight landed in Warsaw in midafternoon the following day. I nervously reached for my papers and joined a line, quickly learning that Poles routinely got on any line they encountered. The early eighties had become the era of shortage, and the people rushed to get on a line, only then bothering to inquire what the line was for.

A well-dressed gentleman gently squeezed my arm and said in a clipped British accent, "Richard, come with me." It was Teddy, who would be my friend until his death from cancer six years later. Teddy had been born into Polish royalty, was educated in England, and flew with the Royal Air Force during the Second World War. Teddy returned to Warsaw and was immediately imprisoned by the emerging Communist government. A sort of fixer for CBS News, Teddy was a survivor.

I never shared my secret, but I listened intently to his stories of intrigue and survival. Teddy would talk of the need for personal strength, and I heard him. Teddy knew everyone in the Communist party. Still, he was followed and harassed, sometimes detained. His personal strength and determination to prevail were an inspiration and put my problems into perspective. His life taught an understated lesson about taking hard blows and moving forward. That Teddy died a few short years before Communism fell in that land of survivors seemed utterly unjust.

On that autumn day in 1981, Teddy hustled me through side doors and past checkpoints. He had my passport stamped on the run. We quickly drove to the CBS News bureau, where a bottle of vodka appeared. We made a few toasts and drank more than a few shots of the vodka. Teddy put his finger to his lips and said, "We will talk later," and we headed back to the airport for the short flight to Gdansk. Once on the tarmac at the Warsaw airport and walking to the ladder of the plane, Teddy turned to me and said, "Never talk indoors. The walls can hear you. So can the government."

We were on the road into Gdansk, a twisting two-lane country street. We took a turn. Ahead were the towers of the vaunted Lenin shipyard rising from the fog. We grew closer and could see graffiti painted on the wall surrounding the shipyard. "What does it say?" I asked Teddy. "It says radio and television lie," he answered. "Radio and television should speak for the people." We stared in silence as a young mother pushed a stroller past the scrawl without a glance.

This was it, the center of the universe. I could not see the scene clearly, because of the fog outside and in my eyes, but I knew what it was. We were driving past a front-page photograph, the sort I had seen so frequently in *The New York Times*, the image of history being made that drew me to Poland in the first place.

I was thriving. My fight was not with

Communism but with myself. I needed to see the world as best I could while I was able to see at all. My neuro-ophthalmologist repeatedly had told me there would always be a fifty-percent chance my eyes would get worse. I was already on the edge, but I was seeing what needed to be seen. My overseas adventures were under way. I was pushing myself hard and, soon enough, recklessly.

Beirut beckoned six months after I left Poland. It was my second trip to the Middle East; the first had come only weeks after my return from Poland. Now, Israel's sudden 1982 war against the PLO spread into southern Lebanon and, to the surprise of many, to the outskirts of Beirut.

My colleague and friend Freddie, a Puerto Rican videotape editor, was standing with me on the check-in line at the TWA ticket counter at JFK International. The line was long and tempers short. I stood clutching my frayed copy of *Zorba the Greek*, which I was rereading. I told Freddie about Zorba, that the fisherman believed we all must dare to live. A swarthy man looked at the equipment cases and noted the CBS News stickers. "Where are you going?" he asked in a hoarse voice. "To Beirut," my good companion said, shrugging. "Good luck," the fellow said as he turned away. A moment passed while my double-take kicked in. "That was Anthony Quinn," I erupted. "Wait here," I shouted, as I began my fruitless search in that crowded terminal.

This was a sign. Zorba said to let go and live. "A man needs a little madness," the Greek advised, warning that otherwise, "he never dares cut the rope and be free." Yes. Cutting the rope was exactly what I was doing. Going for it. How much longer would I be walking and laughing and flying away? Thoughts of cutting the rope danced around much of the flight. The writer's advice applied to a simple fisherman and to my real mission abroad, to live life as if there were no tomorrow. (My mother, of course, might wonder if proving points by taking reckless risks is an appropriate way for a grown-up to live. Probably not, would be my sheepish reply.)

Once in Beirut, I joined a group of journalists traveling north along the Mediterranean coast into Lebanon with the Israeli army. We sat in silence, our eyes wide. My God, this is real, I thought. At that moment, my physical problems seemed small.

We passed the carcasses of Syrian tanks. Everywhere, there were PLO dead, their weapons and live ammunition strewn around them. The fighting went on around us as we headed into the mountains, the Shuf, surrounding the city. The sense of danger was overwhelming. I had been advised at the last minute that crossing the green line separating the Moslem west in Beirut from the Christian east would be dangerous for me because I am a Jew, and there was no accountability in that war zone. Many of the Moslem fighters, including the PLO, were kids with big automatic rifles. I did travel back and forth a bit, and the crossings clearly were the most dangerous part of the stay. Learning to live with fear was hardly new, but this brought it to a new level. I never thought of my physical problems when I was in the Middle East. I had bigger fish to fry. Waking up another day, for example.

I learned a lot about myself that sweaty summer. Winston Churchill wrote of covering the Boer War in South Africa at the turn of the last century, "Nothing is so exhilarating," he wrote, "as to be shot at with no result." Right on. I was shocked that I took to this line of work. A tiny voice inside suggested that if I could survive Lebanon, I could handle MS.

My impaired vision placed me in harm's way all too often. I was on a mission, living

95

too close to the edge and unable to see it. One hot afternoon my camera crew and I were stopped along the Corniche, a beautiful boulevard along the harbor. The tree-lined avenue faced the old U.S. embassy that would fall victim to a car bomb a year later. A PLO patrol checked us out and announced that our papers were not in order.

I crossed the street to speak to their superior, mindful that these were angry young men with big guns and small concerns about killing. The conversation grew heated, and I was waved back across the street. My British camera crew looked at me incredulously and asked how I could yell so loudly when there were guns pointed at my head. "Guns?" I asked. "What guns?" I was out of control, proving nothing but my excessive need to be a boy taking chances. Always, move on. Stay in motion. There will be plenty of time for rest.

For me, functioning as a journalist in the vital arena of critical news symbolized strength. The honest pursuit of truth in an unjust world, the ability to reach across oceans and tell the people what was really going on, was empowering and compensated for the physical weakness I endured. I was doing what I was cut out for. The power to live my way was mine, at least for this moment. I was beating the reaper.

Months later, on the difficult road trip south, heading back into Israel and making our way carefully along the Mediterranean coast, we stopped at Beaufort Castle, an ancient Crusader fort recently recaptured from the PLO by the Israeli army in a bloody battle. We walked to the edge of a towering precipice, looking down on the Latani River, forty kilometers north of the border into Lebanon. The river stretched like ribbon candy. The Golan Heights of Syria stood to our left, the sea to our right. Before us was the patchwork quilt of Israel's kibbutzim.

I stood for a moment with my arms stretched high in the warm sun. Ebullience at having survived the long ordeal overtook me. I was flying, beating the odds and high on my life.

The next winter found me back in Beirut reporting on the brutality of Israel's occupation. It was snowy in the Shuf, and we found ourselves clashing with all parties. I was having more problems with my right leg. One afternoon, I suddenly fell at a checkpoint manned by the United Nations. Automatic weapons of various manufacture and in various hands pointed my way. The incident prompted the first thought that the time had come for me to quit while I was ahead.

Ignoring my instincts, I headed for Central America one year later to cover the war in El Salvador. By now I walked with a subtle limp. I thought life in Salvador was cheap. I had no respect for the government or the rebels. In the Middle East there seemed to be no bullets with our names on them. Here they shot first and asked questions later.

The chip on my shoulder was its own target. If I had flouted danger in the crucible of the Middle East, now I was angry I was in the toilet bowl of Salvador. Risk was large and seemed hardly worth it. Who might I die for? This was Dan Rather's battle in the war of ratings. We were just soldiers. John Blackstone, a correspondent based in San Francisco, and I had lived through Beirut together. We now found ourselves in the hills, inland from beaches blackened by centuries of volcanic ash.

A road had been partially destroyed by the Marxist rebels, and we had to drive on a segment of railroad tracks. We entered a small village with our crew and the shooting suddenly began. We were in the wrong place now. John and I were separated from our crew when we heard the bullets zinging past our heads. John yelled to dive under a car. My right leg collapsed as I tried to join him. I just fell to the ground and rolled under the rear of the vehicle. The ricocheting bullets were everywhere. "What the hell are we doing in this fucking place?" I screamed, conveniently forgetting that I had volunteered for the assignment. I was embarrassed by my need to be reckless. That much I knew.

But I was doing what gave me comfort as a member of the male persuasion. My illness was not going to rob me of any experience I wanted or compromise my masculinity any more than it already had. Covering war and getting shot at is masculine. Right? So I was in these shitholes, falling into ridiculously dangerous situations and diving under parked cars, only seeking the validation of getting shot at, hopefully with no result, to prove that, if absolutely necessary, I could die to live a more fulfilling life.

This made perfect scary sense to me. Putting my life on the line had served if not fed my state of denial about my illness. Trekking through deserts in the Middle East or stumbling through the underbrush of Central America had proved I could do the job, which, of course, meant that I was okay. How bad could my health be if I was dodging bullets? Work had come to define me, so my illness would not.

What had gotten into me? The questions consumed me in the fall of 1983. There has to be a better way to make a living, I thought. I decided to be through with war. I went home and hung up my tin badge. I had hair on my chest now. That others in the news business made careers out of dodging bullets confused me. Why do they run into danger? And what, I wondered, are they running from?

The fact that I was alone in the world weighed heavily. My brief brush with marriage after college had made me single again with a vengeance. Now I was rethinking my solitary existence. It was time to grow up, I thought. Running cannot last forever. Yes, I was alone. And lonely.

six

Enter
Meredith

My thirty-fifth birthday in 1983 had been spent by myself on the eve of yet another trip to Beirut. We flew overnight, arriving in that wretched land in a snowstorm. The assignment turned into a depressing adventure. Beirut was a sad place, and I was sadder, approaching a crossroad and feeling very alone.

An emptiness overtook me in that wretched place. Wet snow covered the mountains outside the city; we were surrounded by deprivation and a life that was bleak. Watching people suffer was just part of the job for the soldiers of news who had spent so much of the previous years as witnesses to a bloody war there. I don't really understand how things became so personal and evocative for me on this trip, but it was at this moment in my life that it suddenly occurred to me that I was a solitary figure. I had no partner, no children. That reality began to gnaw at me. I came home with a new mission on my mind.

My return was to the same quiet apartment in an old brownstone near Riverside Park. The radiator was still hissing, the kitchen faucet dripping as I dropped to an old couch in silence, happy to be home or at least far from the fighting. I sat motionless for days. The plumber needed to be called, bills were overdue, and my life needed change. And not in that order. At that moment, the plumber and creditors took a backseat in my mind. There was a familiar voice in my head.

I had first heard that voice about a year before, in spring 1982. I had been sitting with a colleague, idly listening to the afternoon audio circuits coming into the CBS News headquarters in Manhattan. When videotaped stories were fed into New York from around the world each day, the sound could be heard on speakers located around the newsrooms and studios. We were lounging around the quiet anchor studio, listening as a young woman's warm, throaty voice accompanied a piece on something or other.

"Whose voice is that?" I asked, sitting up

straight. "Meredith Vieira," my pal responded, taken aback by my enthusiastic inquiry. "She is a new correspondent out of Chicago," he went on.

"I am going to marry that woman," I announced without hesitation.

It wasn't until late that year, however, that my path crossed Meredith's. Our first encounter was contempt at first sight. I had gone to the Windy City to cover the windier race for Illinois governor and discovered Meredith in her CBS office. She was wrapped in a blanket, lying on a couch, and watching Looney Tunes cartoons on television. "Very impressive," I remarked as I walked by, adding, "A real journalist, I'd say." Her expletive has been deleted.

Meredith later wandered into my editing room, watched briefly, and casually proclaimed the videotaped story I was producing to be flawed and not worth putting on the air. "If they let Chicago people cover Chicago politics, the story might be more interesting," she said.

I thought she was exceedingly attractive and had a big mouth, both true and highly acceptable qualities. A flirtation and a friendship had been born. I called Meredith a few times after I returned from Beirut, but it wasn't until she came to New York on assignment that our relationship deepened. Our mutual friend, Bonnie, an evening news assistant, went to work, setting us up on a dinner date. We spent the next day walking the city, dining together in the evening. There was suspense and suspicion. We both had pasts.

The attraction between Meredith and me was strong, soon to be consuming. We were both alone and wished our lives were configured differently. Meredith was on the rebound; I was in the grandstands, ready to return to the game. We were temperamentally alike and shared a biting sense of humor.

The critical attitude check came quickly enough. We discussed my health.

The subject was raised on the second date. I had learned long ago to grit my teeth and put the health issue on the table early. Tell the truth. Get on with it. Spare the spectacle. See if the lady runs screaming out of the room. It was not difficult for anyone to figure out that I could not see twenty feet ahead, so the questions always came anyway. A bad reaction would save the price of dessert. Such scenes had played out before. One woman might as well have been told her pants were on fire. She stopped dead in her amorous tracks, scanning the room for a fire exit.

"What do you know about multiple sclerosis?" I asked. Meredith was not reacting. "Do you know what MS means?" I asked. "Yes. It's a magazine, Rich," she answered. Rich became Richard only when the plot thickened. "Is there any chance we can have a serious discussion?" I persisted. And we did.

Meredith did not flinch or reveal any discomfort. She looked me in the eye and asked questions for which, of course, there were no answers. There were pauses and stares into the distance. "I don't care," she finally said. "You have a look of sadness," she added, an observation she has repeated over the years. I think I was more tired than sad and more wary than weary. The subject of my illness was discussed, seemingly endlessly, and picked apart over many dates. It could not be put to rest. "You have to learn to live with ambiguity with this problem," I said. She liked clear lines. I offered a blur. Meredith would have to rack focus and accept the blur, living with soft definition to be with me.

Everything I could say was said over time, but what could I say? Except for seriously impaired eyesight, the full force of the storm had not hit. We were talking about possible

105

outcomes, what might happen down the road. "What is the worst that could happen?" she asked once. "MS could kill me." Meredith paused. "Okay, that is not going to happen," she announced. "What's next?"

Meredith seemed to take her cues from me. And so it went. Endless hypothetical outcomes were proposed. "Could you go blind?" Meredith asked. "Yes." The answer was greeted with a shrug. "Do you think you could end up in a wheelchair?" That gave me pause. "Could?" I asked. "I suppose so. Do I think that will happen? I doubt it."

The wheelchair was where my grandmother sat at the end of her life. My old man was still on his feet. A decade of dealing with MS had hardened my determination that I would cling to my ability to walk. That was a silly assumption, of course, but it worked for me, and apparently I sold it to Meredith. These conversations always seemed to have a "what-if" quality to them. I had the uncomfortable feeling my answers went in one ear and out the other.

This was a large issue for me. I wanted Meredith to know what she was in for. Life with me would be no cakewalk. A wheelchair-free zone did not mean other serious problems would not appear at the door. MS is a progressive disease. I was already practically legally blind, operating with the full knowledge that on any day, the word *legally* might be dropped.

This was a matter of honor with an element of self-protection. Now was the time to spot the weak heart. I was not convinced that anyone could really know what the human reaction to the stress of real problems would be. I have trouble figuring out dinner plans for next Friday night. I was wanting Meredith to predict a long future. We had no certain plans. There were thoughts.

Mostly, Meredith and I laughed and loved and spent wonderful time together, going our separate ways in search of success, returning to each other in celebration. We simply ignored whatever we imagined on the horizon. We did not know what lay ahead. The subject of health seemed unreal because we were too far up the relationship road for the possibilities to click in. Worsening health was framed as tomorrow's problem. There was no car wreck in sight. In the end, Meredith took a leap of faith. "I knew what I wanted," she said later.

A stable, grown-up relationship and a family. So did I. We both had been married to the company for too long. Employers love you to death when it suits them, but they don't kiss back. When your job screws you, there will be no pregnancy. We knew there was more to life than we were getting.

We became an item, an official CBS couple. Our stars were high, though in separate orbits. I went off to China with President Reagan and came home to run CBS News coverage of the 1984 presidential campaign. Meredith moved to New York to become a correspondent on *West 57th*, a new CBS prime-time magazine program. We looked for apartments for her and decided that mine was just fine. We compared notes, though never competed, and we offered each other encouragement and appropriate grief about our respective positions and pieces.

Meredith and I were happy. We lived together in my garden apartment (though she kept forgetting to pay any rent), traveled together to Europe and the Caribbean, and we continued laughing. We had our ups and downs. We were different, an observation as relevant today as it was twenty years ago. We do approach life quite differently. I seem to let nothing get to me. Meredith cares about everything, and she worries and prepares for the worst. I feel that I have seen, even lived the worst.

Meredith had shrugged off my concerns about her attitude toward living with multiple sclerosis in her life, but in the absence of any mutual decision to up the ante in our relationship and go for the gold ring, the worries did not seem real. My worst-case scenarios served no purpose. Her attitude seemed wise because nothing was at stake. I knew Meredith was not calm by nature; her Portuguese heritage and Latin blood give her a tempestuous character and a dangerous temper. Meredith could erupt volcanically and without warning. But once I got used to nitroglycerin stored in the refrigerator, the occasional blowups became no big thing. I just pretended I was back in Beirut. (Things are calmer now. We are getting old.)

Life at the office was more dangerously explosive. The growing cloud formations were barely identifiable on radar, but they were there and moving my way. I was becoming frustrated and angry that CBS News seemed to be serving the Reagan campaign more than viewers and voters. Television loved the president for the pictures the White House served up, and truth was a casualty. Ronald Reagan clearly was the establishment candidate, and we were the establishment and all but endorsed him. I began to feel symptoms of MS creeping over me for the first time in what seemed a long while. It was not a surprise. Stress brings on the problems, and I felt as if I were going to crack.

There were the endless meetings, even confrontations because of my resistance to our style of coverage. Dan Rather was annoyed because I was rocking the boat and inventing headaches. I was upset because I thought he was pandering to popular sentiment and the corporate desire to please the audience.

My emotions about my body and body of work mixed together. I was angry and wanted out. Meredith was riding high at *West 57th*. I felt low, and so I left. The election was over, as was my contract. I left on good terms, with no hard feelings and no commitment ever to return. And no plan. Setting off without a map was a true indication of my frustration. I will show them. I'll flounder. The worry was not the future. The priority was getting away. Ends would be made to meet. Money had been saved. Meredith advised me to go for it, and off we went. To Guadeloupe. That was as far as the itinerary for my life extended.

On our return, I started a bad screenplay

and did freelance work as a producer. I applied to Harvard University and was appointed a Fellow of the Institute of Politics at the Kennedy School of Government. Cambridge became the venue for my self-imposed semester of navel gazing. From the ivory tower I would find myself, sorting out the past and future.

Questions about my anger vexed me. Everyone in the business knew where news was headed. By the mid-1980s, the seriousness, if not the integrity, of the newsroom had been compromised by commercial pressures. Yet I had taken it so personally. I wanted the world to exist my way. Perhaps I sought control, an elusive commodity in my life.

My investment in my work seemed out of proportion and tied to my need to use excellence on the job to compensate for the imperfections in my body. This was pride compensating for shame. Too frequently, I viewed my physical flaws as my own doing, my failure. It was as if illness had been an earned punishment for an aimless, earlier life. That, of course, is an allegation that would be difficult to prosecute in court. But MS had made me feel less of a person. It always has. Larger-than-life status had become the psychological antidote. And perfection in my chosen world of journalism was slipping out of my grasp.

My life was under my own microscope at Harvard. So was the relationship with Meredith. Everything was questioned, including our future. Meredith's regular visits to Cambridge were not always smooth and easy. We were in different places. Without question, we had fallen in like. But was it love? Did love even exist? To me, love seemed underwhelming and overrated, a 1930s movie concept without lasting power.

The many questions about our futures were on the table. We both sensed that decision time was fast approaching. Harvard would soon end for me and something else would fill the void. We knew each of us wanted a family with children, but it was not clear if it should be with each other.

I did not want to repeat the mistake of my failed marriage. The first time around, there seemed to be diminishing compatibility. My wife and I had never reached a consensus about having children or about how we wanted to live our lives. The diagnosis of MS had come in those few years of marriage, but it was still not clear to me how much illness played into our parting. I did know that sickness in a marriage tests the commitment and places enormous stress on the bond.

Preparing to leave Cambridge, I was invited to return to CBS News. At the same time, another offer came from *Frontline*, an acclaimed national documentary series produced for PBS by the public station in Boston. Each had its appeal. A decision to remain in Massachusetts would certainly mean the end of my relationship with Meredith.

I went home to New York. The trip back was easy. I wanted to grow up and settle down. I wanted to have kids before I hit forty. That was an arbitrary but real goal and only a few years away. And I needed the safety net of a long-term relationship. Mostly, I admitted to myself that I really cared about Meredith.

Still, I wasn't sure if marriage was a necessary part of the equation. Why couldn't we have children and just skip the marriage part? That plan was discussed at high volume on the beach at St. Bart's as 1985 turned into 1986. Meredith was appalled and offended, squelching the idea before the speech had ended. Actually, she seemed hurt. I just grew silent.

Multiple sclerosis and relationships did not seem to mix, at least not for me. I was so defensive and so put off by the illness that I projected my doubts and fears onto other people. The more aware I was of the ticking bomb in my body, the greater my skittish withdrawal from the prospect of a serious relationship. My health had become an issue with women before. "I just cannot handle it," one said to me as she got up out of her chair and left. Why would I go back for more of that? My lack of trust in humanity on this issue was not reassuring.

Meredith traveled to Bangkok on a story about Vietnam-era expatriates, and I sat in the hotel room we were occupying while my apartment was being renovated. I was now a senior producer with Rather, another tour of duty, this time overseeing international news. I was furiously reading scripts and taking international phone calls, going to meetings and recutting stories in what felt like a round-the-clock job. Meredith was on her way home. One day, at the end of January 1986, to my utter surprise and on legs weakened more by apprehension than by MS, I walked into a fancy jewelry store. Debating whether to rob the place or buy a ring, I swallowed hard and pulled out a wallet, rather than a weapon.

My questions had not been put to rest, the big question to Meredith not yet popped.

When Meredith returned, we went to dinner at a fancier establishment than usual. We had the requisite conversation turning to disagreement about an irrelevant tidbit of CBS gossip. And then it was time. I mumbled something about shrimp cocktail sauce being thicker than water. "I love you," I said to my astonishment, and the ring was proffered. "Would you marry me?"

Meredith was shocked and answered in the affirmative, obviously before coming to her senses. The deed was done and we have never looked back. With all of the rocks over which we have tripped, stumbled, and fallen, the commitment is strong. It had to be, in ways we could not anticipate. I paid the bill that night. In a sense, Meredith has been paying it since.

Having children was a foregone conclusion. It came close to our reason for being together. Despite my family's neurological history, conventional wisdom continued to deny a genetic link with MS. My mother's words after my diagnosis was made three decades earlier echoed faintly. "I never would have had children if I had known they would have MS," she had cried out in a moment of high emotion, shocked that MS had showed up in the house yet again. I would hear those words again down the road. "I never would have had children if I had thought they might get MS," Meredith has said in fear and frustration, though the thought of that woman without children does not ring true.

It is too soon to know genetic truth, but for all our talk, there is no preparing for illness. The guilt of parents who feel culpable for passing along illnesses they did not know they carried or did not realize could be passed on yields little but emotional pain. They had their children, however, and here we are. Let's all get used to it. A troubled life beats having no life at all.

That is the point. By telling me that she would have forgone bearing children, if only she had known, my mother unwittingly labeled my life a tragedy. It was only a cry of the moment, but she might as well have told me that she wanted to spare me the pain of existing. I, of course, think I have had a great life, and it ain't over yet. I have traveled the world, covered history as it was made, loved passionately and well. Am I supposed to feel sorry for myself? I don't think so.

There is no denying the pain I have felt from illness. Yet all things must be put in perspective. The upside of my life more than compensates for the downside. I could be happier, to be sure, but I am happy.

Whether we suffered from denial or were duped by docs who did not know that of which they spoke, events played out smoothly enough. June 1986 was a happy time. We were on our way, though to where, we could not have imagined.

We had a lovely wedding in the courtyard behind our newly renovated apartment, catered by an old friend and attended by family and colleagues. Rain had dominated the weather all week, but the June sky was clear, the sun bright on the day we were wed. Meredith was beautiful, radiant and beaming. She looked happier than I had seen her or would see her again in years to come.

I do not believe Meredith fully realized what she was getting into. Forces in motion tend to stay in motion, though, and we were caught up in our momentum. Meredith defied her customary caution. The disease process did prove relentless. There was to be an inevitability to our life together, a script already written but unread.

seven

Reentry

My return to CBS immediately pointed me toward physical trouble and professional disaster. Nothing had changed. The place was as tense as when I left. Stress sets off neurological landmines, and I was climbing back into the pressure cooker. I came back to New York and CBS News in great physical condition. Symptoms of MS were few, and I felt good. That lasted for a week or two. I had been running as much as ten miles a day. Now I would be running the gauntlet. My weight was down. My spirits were soon to follow.

The physical toll from reentry came instantly. When I awoke the morning after my return to the Rather news, my voice was hoarse and very hard to hear. Talking was uncomfortable, listening to me worse. That failing voice, later diagnosed as dystonia, was probably the product of a neurological process related to MS in a time of stress. So I was told. Was this a harbinger of what lay ahead? I did not know and had no particular confidence that any doctor did either.

Whenever a neurologist told me that some new problem might be related to MS, I checked for my wallet. The catch-all pronouncement of dystonia was based on assumption that could not disguise the lack of certain knowledge behind it. A shrug and decision to just move on was the only response that made sense to me. The more questions I asked about my voice, the more mute the doctor became.

I knew I had become a walking Rube Goldberg contraption, with one problem invariably leading to another because of the stress multiple sclerosis foists on the systems of the body. And new symptoms were only a matter of time. There were no answers or predictions, no prognosis that held water. Talking to neurologists felt like a kind of pantomime, dancing without music.

Multiple sclerosis is a mystery affliction. Symptoms are treated with no real understanding of causes. There are no certain outcomes, only a journey without the map. Religious faith was in short supply, but a naïve faith in my ability to prevail stayed strong. I was going to win.

This was 1986. The palace guard at CBS had changed, replaced by cowboys in white hats who turned out to be the well-disguised bad guys. These were bottom-liners, suits who insisted on unreasonable profits, far above those generated by most businesses. My voice had a menacing tone, which I cultivated and played to the hilt. I wanted to believe that my growl cast me as the threatening character I longed to be, building newsroom bombs and fomenting revolution. I became part of the cabal that was going to return serious, hard news to its rightful place.

As if anyone in trans-Hudson America cared or even knew it was missing. I know now that my self-righteous zeal was intimately tied to my illness. As my physical strength was diminished from the multiple sclerosis, my determination to adopt strong positions and act with power was increasing. I was dealing psychologically with a chronic illness, in part, by flexing my work muscles. I was seeking to control a life that knew no such thing by trying to impose my clout in the newsroom.

That is not so unusual. Clout can be a strong currency, buying faith in the future.

My friend Don suffers from Crohn's disease, an ailment of the digestive tract. The greater his physical difficulties over the years, the more committed he became and the harder he worked. Don's position as a senior executive at the National Endowment for the Humanities has become his crusade, due in no small part to his physical ailment. So, too, my job became my crusade.

Soon I was engaged in battles over hard leads, budgets, and staffing. Management began laying off hundreds of employees. At that moment, the lives of my comrades carried more urgency than my health. This was signature denial. I simply identified those hurting more than I and made them the issue. Perhaps I needed to ride the white charger so that no one would notice my emerging limp.

My anger at the television news business had returned, and by 1987, it was clear to me that I should not have returned to my old haunts. In March 1987, after the body count was completed, I penned an essay for the op-ed page of *The New York Times*, entitled "Morrow to Mediocrity." The piece accused the CBS chairman, Laurence Tisch, of eviscerating the news division with layoffs and dragging it down. Dan Rather signed the essay, though all knew that I had written it. That fact had been leaked to the papers to embarrass the anchorman. "Cohen is committing suicide," a vice president said at the time.

Publicly criticizing the company CEO, beating him over the head in the newspaper of record, cannot be considered a sound career move. But my anger at my job was also well-camouflaged rage at my illness. I was flailing in my fury, internalizing all the pressures from the outside, taking the betrayals personally and mixing them with anger at my slowly crumbling body.

The end for me was drawing near. The 1988 presidential campaign had heated up by late 1987. I was slated to manage the political coverage. At a cordial breakfast in November, I discussed the coming race with Howard Stringer, then the President of CBS News, adding that I would leave CBS following the election. This time, I said, there would be no round-trip ticket. Howard scoffed. "You won't leave, Richard." He laughed. "You'll never leave." Wrong. I barely made it to Super Tuesday.

George Herbert Walker Bush was vice president and wanted to be Reagan's successor in the oval office. In a crowded field of candidates, Bush was the story going into the Iowa caucuses because of unanswered questions about his role in the controversial Iran-Contra affair. The *CBS Evening News* was profiling all the candidates but zeroed in on the Bush record on Iran-Contra. In a great moment of political theater, we confronted the vice president live on the evening news, forcing him to defend his role in the illegal scheme to funnel money to anticommunist rebels in Nicaragua by selling arms to Iran.

We ran a tough report raising questions about Bush's role, how much he knew and what advice he had given President Reagan. That story was followed by an unprecedented nine-minute live interview, an epic by evening news standards. The interview quickly disintegrated into a debate, if not a brawl. The vice president accused us of misleading him about the subject matter of our report, suggesting that I had been dishonest. The confrontation touched off a national debate about the propriety of what had happened. Many newspapers and magazines seemed to buy the vice president's line that we had set a trap. *Time* put the story on its cover, labeling the incident, "The ambush that failed."

The Bush claim was wrong, and I was right at home, angry at the Bush campaign, disappointed with the press corps, and feeling very much the victim. It felt all too familiar. My pattern of anger was long established. I believed the Bush interview was defensible as journalism and said so to everyone. I also felt that Dan Rather had made mistakes in his conduct of the interview, having crossed a line and appearing to be disrespectful to a man none of us much respected. I said as much to the Des Moines *Register*. My death wish had played out. Dan turned on me, and I soon departed CBS.

A long soul-searching process followed. Much of it took place as I was shaving each morning. Looking in the bathroom mirror, squinting and wondering just who was staring at me so intently, the linkage between job difficulties and illness became clear. I was not a victim. Nor did I want to be. Victim status embodies all that I reject about the struggles of life. The challenge is to live and function well under all circumstances, including those never anticipated, like illness.

These sense-seeking seminars before the mirror became an exercise in taking responsibility and facing reality. I was unhealthy in body but alive, and I needed a new venue for proving my strength. *Time* invited me to join the magazine as a contributor. That sounded like a start on a new road. Then came a breathtaking breakthrough toward achieving my fondest dream. On an early June morning, as fathers all over America celebrated their special day, Meredith walked downstairs, smiling. "Happy Father's Day," she said softly, "Dad."

Meredith was pregnant, although not for the first time. Three miscarriages had come early in previous pregnancies, causing great pain and upset amid the clamor and chaos of our CBS years. Meredith's miscarriages were devastating. They really were *our* miscarriages. They had been *our* pregnancies.

The miscarriages had occurred suddenly, before I could even process the idea of impending parenthood in my head, let alone find a way to be involved. I had stood on the sidelines and watched in mute wonder as new life was proclaimed, and I listened in horror as the faint and fading heartbeat went silent. I found myself feeling more helpless than I had ever felt before. My response to the miscarriages, the tears and pure pain, were in stark contrast to my reactions to the problems at work and my own difficulties. There was nothing I wanted in my life more than children. The pregnancy problems had begun in 1986 and went on for close to two years. There would be more losses, including twins after our first child was born. Then the problem disappeared.

In the summer of 1988, we traipsed nervously to the obstetrician's office for the ritual soundings of life. We were three months into the pregnancy, at the conclusion of the first trimester. We should see that heartbeat, even hear it, through the magic of ultrasound. The indication of healthy life, which we had seen only briefly in previous attempts, would provide confirmation that all was well. The moment was decisive and exhilarating. Our fortunes had changed.

Benjamin Edwin Cohen arrived in February of 1989, wide-eyed and alert. "Congratulations," the attending pediatrician quipped after examining him one day later. "You have a healthy, three-month-old child." Ben's neck was unusually strong. He could hold his head up straight. Ben rode my shoulder to parties when he should have been home in bed, and rode my back on long walks up Broadway, which was just fine. We took him everywhere. Ben would stare silently at everything that passed us, dogs and buses, and the varied exotic types who frequented the Upper West Side near Columbia University.

Ben was the reason Meredith and I had

taken the leap and landed together. He filled a hole in our lives. I changed instantly. My perspective and priorities shifted and grew. "My career seems very far away," I told Meredith. "It is far away, stupid," she answered. "Now it's just a job." I was beginning work with Bill Moyers on a PBS documentary about the press. There would be occasional trips to California, numerous ones to Washington. But my wanderlust was missing. I just wanted to give Ben his five a.m. bottle, my only such opportunity, sharing a bed with a nursing mother.

Meredith had talked CBS into a seven-month maternity leave from *West 57th*, a broadcast to which she would never return. Life at home was fun, work relaxed in the preproduction phase. But there were the stresses and sleeplessness of first-time parents. I was up a lot at night, if only in solidarity with Meredith, who had taken to being a mother as if she had done it all before. She did not need my help to tend to Ben, as she never tired of reminding me. "You are a mom," I would answer. "You can do everything yourself, one hand tied behind your back."

My identity was changing. Ben was far too young to call me "Dad," but that is what I had longed to hear. Not journalist or producer. Just Dad. We bought a car. We traveled out of the city on weekends, throwing Ben into his car seat and heading to the old house we had bought in the country. For the first time in years, I felt like everything had clicked into place. I felt normal.

That didn't last for long. I began to be more tired than usual, which surprised me because I was sleeping well, and the hard work of the documentary had yet to begin. Something was off.

"How fast are you going?" I asked Meredith one Saturday morning as we traveled my highway of fog, heading north along the Hudson. "The speed limit," she answered. "I can't read the big green exit signs," I said, with obvious concern in my voice. "Slow down when we come to another one," I said, sitting up straight. A while later, the car slowed slightly. "There is an exit coming," Meredith said softly.

There was little traffic to negotiate, and we slowed to a crawl. "My god, I can't begin to make out what the sign says," I stammered. "Where are we?" Meredith seemed shocked. "Cold Spring," she said. My eyesight had been stable for thirteen years. This is not happening, I thought.

Everything had been so wrong, then so right in my life. Thoughts raced through my mind: I had found the religion of family and was paying the price . . . I had traded a job for a child . . . perhaps a career . . . no good deed goes unpunished. I loved Ben with all my heart, and this was my baptism into fatherhood. There had been an uncharacteristic calm to our existence. That was sailing out the window. We had a peaceful home, the sense that we had settled in for the long haul. The keel, finally, had become even. A wave of anger was all that I could feel now.

The neuro-ophthalmologist confirmed the loss of vision and sent me to a different neurologist, who ordered an MRI. There were new lesions on my already stressed-out brain. I was ordered into the hospital. Before going, I had gone downstairs at Channel Thirteen to discuss my situation with Bill Moyers. Bill did not know I had MS. I hated telling people the facts of my life. They always are shocked and do not know what to say. So I end up doing the talking myself, sometimes tap-dancing. Usually, they have nothing to say. Bill was different. "Richard, your health is all that is important here," he said calmly, "not the documentary. This is only television. It doesn't matter. Don't forget that." I smiled. "I will be back," I told him.

Into the hospital I went, where I was

hooked to an IV and began receiving industrial-strength steroids. Dr. Frankenstein dreamed up this therapy. Anyone who is not a mess going into the hospital for intensive steroid treatments is a maniac on departure. I spent almost two weeks taking decreasing doses of the drug orally, weaning myself off the poison. Steroids made me fat and crazy. My mood swings were wild. Feelings of well-being turned to depression precipitously, a journey as quick as crossing the street, which was considerably riskier now. Trying to cope, to put the threatening changes into perspective, seemed impossible. I was too wired. By the end of summer, 1989, I would be forty pounds heavier, and miserable.

The despair I felt was new to me. The constant feeling of weakness kept me from the gym. The weight stayed on, and my self-image suffered. I kept thinking I had to get over it and on with my life. My talks with myself made little difference. Ben and Meredith were my only source of pleasure.

I hit bottom hard on a weekend in the country. A sleepless night drove me downstairs to read. At dawn, my head began to ache. I thought little of it and found aspirin in the kitchen. I rejoined my book, nervously realizing that the pain in my head was growing sharper, joined by a dull throbbing that came in waves. This was a new experience. I climbed the stairs and headed into the bedroom. Lying next to Meredith, I tried to relax and only grew tense.

Pain usually is a stranger to multiple sclerosis. The illness generally is characterized by pain's polar opposite, the loss of sensation. By now, numbness was my constant companion. This new pain threw me. Where was it coming from? I lay there, aware that the dagger in my skull was now twisting. Meredith was awakened by the groans. "My head is in a vise," I cried out. The pain was so intense I was losing my grip. "I've got to call the doctor," I said to no one in particular. My neurologist returned the call at 6:30 a.m. I was in tears. "Go to Columbia," he instructed. "You're not a complainer. I know this is real. I will meet you there." We had a two-hour drive ahead. We threw Ben in the back and left.

And there we were, careening down the New York State Thruway, crying baby in the back, hysterical father in the front. All I could think was, I am going to die. I've worked so hard for so long to live with this shit, and this is it. I was crying wildly. "Pull over, Meredith," I suddenly shouted. "Please pull off the road. I am going to be sick."

Meredith hit the brakes, swerving onto the shoulder. Before the station wagon could stop, my window was down, my head extended out, and I was vomiting powerfully out the window. The car stopped with a jerk. My head dropped into my arms. And then there was nothing. The pain was gone.

My neurologist never could explain the mysterious event. It sounded like a migraine headache, he said, though there was no history of any kind of headaches. I chose to view the brutal episode as just an unexplained event. That is what life had become to me.

There was always something else around the bend. Even as I was beginning to appreciate personal responsibility, my awareness of serendipity was acute. There was much in my body that could not be explained. Why should this be any different?

I kept coming back to my loss of control, as if that power had been there at all for the more than fifteen years that MS had been stalking me. No neurologist had helped me. Of that I was convinced. They only listed what was not understood and what they thought was happening. And that was offered with such authority. My raspy voice, well, probably MS. The incredible exploding head? Probably related to MS. Please. My disdain for television by now was matched only by my contempt for doctors. Nobody was in charge here, was all I could think. And the slope down the mountain was getting steeper.

eight

A Seismic Shift

At last, September arrived. Air was invisible again. The miserable, hot summer of 1989, mercifully, was ending. This had been my season of living dangerously. The emotional freefalls from the flare-ups of MS had matched the physical devastation. Steroids had thrown fuel on the fire but were but a bad memory now. The horrid drugs were long gone and out of my body. I had moved from growing fat and crazy to just being fat.

Now my neurologist was talking me into participating in a clinical trial of Botox, a derivative of botulism toxin. Cosmetic applications for Botox had yet to be discovered, but doctors thought it might restore the faltering voice that had turned harsh immediately on my return to CBS three years earlier. All I knew now was that a very long needle would be stuck into my throat.

The thin needle pierced the skin, entering my throat and penetrating the larynx. "Is there any end to this stuff?" I asked myself as I lay back with a pillow beneath my neck. A silent "Why me?" came roaring into my head as a dangerous follow-up. The camel's back was weakening. Why me? That question never was posed out loud in my family. There is no answer. The inquiry serves no one. That plaintive cry reflects weakness. No, no, no.

I had learned that years earlier when I had developed a hernia on one side of my groin. That problem was not uncommon for guys. A surgical repair was required. Feeling beleaguered and tired of the MS I had then suffered for only five years, I allowed that two-word, self-serving query to pass my lips. In a conversation with my old man, I suggested that everything bad seemed to happen to me. *Bam.* "You are talking like a professional asshole," my dad snapped back. Message received.

Beyond the pinprick of entry, there was no pain to the Botox injection. "Have there been any casualties?" I had asked the neurologist. "Just a broken ankle," he answered. "A lady got so scared that she jumped off the table and landed in the emergency room." That sounded funny enough, at least until the procedure began.

A gagging reflex came on swiftly, and the needle just popped out of my neck. The weapon attacked my throat once more, only to jump out again. The gagging could not be controlled. "That was fun," I snarled, grimacing in discomfort. "Let me guess," I said. "You are going to do that again." The red-haired maniac in whites just smiled and nodded his head up and down. The silver bullet was fired again, finally remaining in place. It was determined soon enough that I had received the wrong dosage. My voice now went silent, erasing my ability to even speak audibly.

I very quietly went back to work on the PBS documentary *Illusions of News*, which I was directing and producing for Bill Moyers. I headed to the cutting room, intent on saving the film. Through all of my distractions of the long summer, the program was shaping up as a disaster, resting mostly on the cutting room floor. "Richard, you have a powerful story to tell," Moyers would plead, "and you are not telling it." Bill was right, and I knew this hour of television was in jeopardy.

I was demoralized. My health had been heading south on an extended trip, and it was taking my confidence along for the ride. My usual problems with structure were at work, growing only more complicated by my growing confusion about treating the symptoms of MS. I found myself in yet another editorial meeting with Moyers. I bit my lip, cleared my throat, and tried to speak.

No words were coming out. Helplessness had set in. My physical problems, once again, were beyond my ability to control, a situation I had faced before but never grown used to. "What," Bill practically screamed. "I can't hear you. What are you saying?" He shook his head in frustration. I whispered almost silently that I would struggle to fix the film. This was not a high point for me, only an endurance test. I had come to believe I could handle anything short of a dirt blanket. Sheer determination brought the beast under control, along with the patient prodding of a sympathetic boss. You have to want something awfully badly to win under these circumstances, I thought.

Meredith was having her own problems at CBS. Her work on *West 57th* had won glowing reviews, and the folks at CBS News just liked her. One executive she had impressed was Don Hewitt, the creator and executive producer of *60 Minutes*, who offered her the slot vacated by Diane Sawyer, who had already left for ABC News.

Meredith was excited by the prospect but had reservations about the travel demands. She took four-month-old Ben to lunch with Hewitt to make a point. Here was her priority, sitting in diapers next to Don at a fancy restaurant. Meredith was a very happy mommy and didn't intend to give that up for anything. Work part-time, work at home, Hewitt responded. Bring Ben to the office. We will get a crib. Hewitt made it sound easy.

It ain't necessarily so. Meredith could not make her peace with her vacillating new boss. Hewitt's commitment to Meredith ran an inch deep. She never reconciled the dual responsibilities and competing loyalties to family and job. Leaving Ben at home, even for a routine day at the office, was difficult. The necessary travel for the job never grew less painful. Meredith headed to Romania for a week to shoot a story about orphans. All she could think about was the child back home whom she had orphaned by her departure. I was home — Meredith and I had made a pact never to travel for work at the same time — but that did not count. I did not qualify as a mother.

When Meredith returned from Romania,

Ben would not so much as acknowledge her presence. She had to be punished for taking that long voyage without him. I was newly empowered as a father, however, having survived my time alone with Ben quite nicely. My view of myself was changing. I no longer missed the big time. I liked being with my kid. Secretly, I loved Meredith's short stint in purgatory. Change had arrived. Parenthood suited me. No disease could touch that.

Miraculously, I had fixed my documentary and recovered my voice. Neither had seemed a sure thing. We were in the final stages of editing the film in the neighborhood, and Ben would get packed into his stroller and head with me each day to the editing room. Once there, he would lie on a clean sheet on the floor and amuse himself with various toys. My recent vision loss had not much corrected itself, but I could see that Ben enjoyed the floor, and I the film. *Illusions of News* was broadcast on PBS to critical acclaim shortly before Thanksgiving. The documentary won an Emmy and a John Foster Peabody Award.

My life with MS had now been under way for more than sixteen years. Coping with multiple sclerosis by now had become the long march, surviving and trying to shield the important people in my life from having to deal with it any more than was necessary. Managing illness was routine, a day-to-day affair. Exacerbations were more challenging than they were upsetting. MS patients learn to wait patiently for trouble, recognizing inevitability but in no hurry to suffer.

By the close of 1989, I was still shaky on my feet and desperately out of shape, still suffering from poststeroid bloat. A *60 Minutes* friend told me about a spa in California, where guests hiked in the mountains and were starved to death in the lodge. That had some appeal, and arrangements were made. The morning I was to fly it was hard even to walk. My right leg was almost buckling as I headed for JFK. On the ground in Venice, a bizarre Bohemian beach community south of Los Angeles, I tried walking on the beach with a cousin. The soft sand cushioned my few falls. *How am I going to hike in the mountains?* I wondered. But I figured that the problem would increase or decrease soon enough, perhaps even go away.

This exacerbation, though, was to inaugurate a new phase of my life. I was crossing a line and would not return. Hiking in the Santa Monica Mountains with Faye Dunaway was not so bad. It was dragging my leg and stumbling, eventually falling

140

into a gully, and breaking my right foot and writhing in pain that was terrible. My hiking companion of the moment went for help.

As I lay on my back I squinted, looking into the blazing sun. A vulture was hovering, circling overhead. "Get out of here, you son of a bitch," I yelled, though I knew I had turned a corner. My illness, so long centered in my eyes, was moving firmly south to my legs. More would follow. My calm felt different from numbness. I felt. I accepted.

That incident gave evidence to the sad fact that hiking across any rough terrain on a leg seriously weakened by multiple sclerosis should be and would be out of the question. And there was little but tough climbing before me in my life. My mission, as always, had been to prove that I was fit and right as rain, that I could still do things with the best of them. I could not pull it off, however, and the time to learn that lesson was as high in the sky as the desert sun.

I broke a foot twice more in the coming weeks, my left as I walked down a road with Ben in a backpack, sending him sprawling. My right foot went, again, as I stepped on a piece of firewood on Christmas Eve. Ben's header into a mud puddle and my long, painful crawl in freezing temperatures back to the house from a dark garage told me something had to change. I could not keep pressing my luck.

"Stop running," the orthopedist advised. "You are blind, and you can't find your footing. Your legs are unstable and the ligaments are stretched. Your equilibrium is shot," he said. "Get it? You are a disaster waiting to keep happening. Stop running." Stop running? Easier said than done. Running was an important and powerful metaphor for my life. I can never stop running, but I did stop jogging.

With braces on both ankles, I joined a gym. The terrain of the treadmill had no charm. Climbing on a stair machine instead of a rugged mountainside brought no aesthetic satisfaction. The zenlike quality of the outdoor jog was missing and missed. But I was in a survival mode, desperately trying to preserve hard exercise as an option in my life. An experiment in common sense was under way. I wasn't so lucky on the work front. I embarked on a project doomed to certain failure, a public affairs program that tilted so sharply to the left that the content slid off. I was working on a PBS pilot on public issues, financed by a political radical, which showed no common sense on my part. I knew this project was going nowhere. I wondered if I was headed anywhere myself.

Our apartment was growing small even as we knew the family would grow only larger. Two men with guns broke into our building and yelled through our locked front door that they were going to kill us. We looked at each other and nodded. It was time to leave. Meredith and I grabbed Ben and moved out of New York City in 1990, heading up the Hudson.

The luxury of a house replaced the confines of an apartment. Houses have stairs, my new venue for falling. New Yorkers take one step out of the city and instantly call their surroundings the country. There were trees and hills overlooking the river, close enough to country for us but suburban in reality.

That was a life decision and a change of venue that would bring profound change to my relationship with Meredith. A life outside the big city, with every destination of importance spread around a large area, would present a test I could not pass. Yet I was the one pushing to leave New York. "Conehead," as my friend Mark likes to call me, "I don't know how you are going to live out there. You have everything you need at your fingertips here in the city. You can't drive anymore. This is going to put a burden on Meredith."

Mark was one of those guys with strong common sense. I hated that. "You are just an actor," I would tell him when I knew he had a point. "Leave me alone." My determination to leave would not crack. A life away from New York would be good for the kids we would bring into the world. New surroundings did not sound so bad for us, either.

I was back in denial about myself, somehow convinced that I could beat the 'burbs. The logistics would be difficult, the burden on others real, but the change just felt right. MS was slowly overtaking me, but I was going to win, and there was no denying my resolve. My neurologist and I sat, surrounded by his earnest entourage, garbed in white coats and wearing studied faces. We were talking in the sparse examining room where the doctor holds court. "This man is in deep denial," the doctor casually announced in no context to his acolytes. "I deny that," I shot back. The guy must have figured I was deaf as he droned on, just looking through me.

The weak attempt at humor obscured my flash of anger that this man would so dismissively deconstruct my carefully choreographed defense against the psychological ravages of multiple sclerosis. Of course, the neurologist was correct about my denial. But he did not understand its evolution. I was selectively ignoring limitations. I knew what I was up against. My life was changing. I wanted to keep up with the change in my body by fighting the word *no.*

Resistance came from strange places. Few people understood the struggle. Individuals in my life, whether in a white coat, an apron, or a faded denim jacket, demonstrate a peculiar need to judge my denial. The crime draws quick responses, usually tilting to the negative. "You shouldn't do that," a friend exclaimed when I said I wanted to hike up a ski mountain one summer day. "You won't make it to the top," he predicted. Really. So what? What this guy imagined might happen was beyond me.

Stopping, perhaps. Possibly even turning around. Imagine that. People seem threatened by denial. Maybe they are intimidated by the ability to go forward in hard times because they imagine they could not.

My problem has long been that I must grapple with the demons of others, even while sparring with my own. One friend tells me I take too many chances. Another announces that I do not know what is good for me. "You go to the gym too much," my father told me a few years ago. "You can push yourself too hard, you know." There are those who kill with concern.

I check out the word *denial* in my own, highly personal dictionary, published and read exclusively by me. My definition: denial (*noun*): 1. a refusal to acknowledge someone else's truth. 2. feeling good to make things good. 3. assuming things will work out when no one else does; stupid denial (*noun*): assuming things will work out when there is no chance.

Our move out of the city seemed to have an element of both good and stupid denial written all over it. I knew to expect difficulties but chose to ignore their probable impact in search of a greater good for the family. My loss of independence was immediate and became an instant burden for Meredith.

The city is a great leveler. Individuals become equals on the streets. Blind men and women in wheelchairs can negotiate the pavement, maintaining their independence. Walking is a signature activity of New York. So is riding public transportation. Errands are everyone's daily responsibility. In our new place, destinations were spread wide.

Suburbia is the land of the automobile, and I am too blind to drive. The ability to drive had pulled away and left me in the dust almost fifteen years earlier.

When we moved into our house, Meredith went straight to the car. She was now in the transit business. She would have to be the one to pilot kids to playdates with friends, to violin lessons, and sports practises. I was to be the permanent copilot, without even an occasional turn at the controls. The passenger seat was to be another prison.

This new living arrangement and ferry service marked a shift in roles away from the traditional. Life was lopsided. I was powerless to do my share, to drive to a party, or to go to the store to purchase that loaf of bread or bottle of wine. Sightlessness is weakness; weakness unmasculine; unmasculine, what a man cannot bear. Apparently, we men are what we drive.

I did not drive myself crazy with my frustration, but the impatient longing for wheels has never gone away. This kind of adjustment did not come easy. I knew what I was getting into with the move out of the city. Meredith did not want to leave New York. Now she feels at home and I want to go back to Babylon. Life may not be what we might have chosen for ourselves. We did it for the children.

By late 1990, Meredith's life at *60 Minutes* was almost unbearable. She was bringing all the tension and unhappiness home, where it mixed easily with my own black mood. We were not the happiest of families. The guilt of spoon-feeding stress to our child only joined the dark emotions swirling around the kitchen, anyway. Something was going to give.

Flexibility for Meredith at *60 Minutes* seemed to have vanished, apparently for good. Work at home? Sure. But when Meredith's backroom office at CBS was empty, the executive producer was agitated. Where was she? Why wasn't she in the office? This isn't working. Meredith's office suddenly was moved up front, next to and in plain sight of Hewitt's door. The man was relentless. He began to question the quality of Meredith's work. He was punishing her for putting family first.

The tension only increased. Meredith was now a second-class citizen. The ugly situation did not make sense. Her stories on *60 Minutes* were well received, even acclaimed by television critics. All but the executive producer believed in Meredith and said as much. When Meredith chose to bring Ben to the office with her, which was not often, discomfort filled the air. Ben became known in the halls as the Baby Jesus. His very presence fought the *60 Minutes* culture. When Ben cried one day, Mike Wallace emerged from his office, loudly yelling, "Get that fucking kid out of here." I thought Meredith was going to collapse under the weight of old men tap-dancing on her head.

The poison kept spreading in our home, by now infecting all of us deeply. Even the dog looked nervous. There was tension, high-voltage electricity in the air, and we were all getting shocks. Meredith had become a whipping girl for the old boys, the *60 Minutes* white male power structure. They seemed to revel in her misery. For Hewitt, it seemed like kicking a dog. If misery loves company, the stress only increased my MS problems. Numbness and weakness became regular visitors.

Meredith was not altogether blameless. She had insisted in newspaper interviews on presenting her job loyalties as holding second place to her child. She was waving red in front of the bull, rubbing her boss's face in her family values. Meredith paid no homage to her masters, kissed no hindquarters. She showed no regard for how her keepers viewed the world they so fiercely controlled. Meredith was proud not to play politics, an exploding Pyrrhic victory in the end.

Meredith and I suffered from the same condition, a swollen notion of our abilities to control our own worlds. This was less from arrogance than the high-minded belief that our way was the best way for each of us. We conceded little ground and fought losing battles. Meredith was born to die at *60 Minutes*, and she did it in style.

When Meredith became pregnant with Gabe, she did not immediately confide in the father figures on Fifty-seventh Street, home to CBS News. With her history of miscarriages, this automatically became a high-risk pregnancy, and her obstetrician told her to stay off airplanes and out of pressure situations. When Hewitt called one Saturday to send her to Paris on a sudden assignment, Meredith gulped and told him her story. The ice age set in. Raising young guys simply held more appeal for her than fighting old guys who thought life began at seven o'clock, six central, on Sunday nights.

Meredith's choice had been made. The decision had been easy, the relief strong. Putting family first was unequivocal. Meredith's decision to choose children over the fountain of fame took enormous guts. That is Meredith. The commitment to family, a determination to be true to self, can see a person through any crisis, including illness. Meredith is always there. She decided what mattered to her most — her family — and went there.

Meredith's troubles resonated with many Americans, prompting a debate about priorities, children, and careers. One cover of a national tabloid carried a photo of Meredith and Ben, with a headline that screamed, YOUR BABY OR YOUR JOB. A more dignified op-ed piece in *The New York Times* addressed the issue, carrying the byline and compromise view of fellow journalist and mother Linda Ellerbee. Don Hewitt did need and deserve a full-time correspondent, she said. On the other hand, she pointed out, "Corporations don't always keep score. Children do. . . . I admire Meredith Vieira for not being afraid to put her career on hold in order to be a mother."

Gabriel Anthony Cohen came to live with us in August 1991. Gabe was the product of a tough labor and difficult birth, a hard day's night. Labor began late in the day and ended at dawn. A 250-pound anesthesiologist crawled onto the table in the delivery room and leaned over Meredith, literally pushing Gabe out of his mother's swollen belly.

To this day, Gabriel likes to do things in his own distinctive way. The boy is listening to a drummer I do not always hear. Gabe would end up a middle child, as was his father. My identification with his family position is complete. Gabe is learning that a kid stuck in between oldest and youngest can feel misplaced in the chronological family sandwich.

The middle child watches the oldest getting the privileges, the youngest the coddling. The kid in the middle is left to look in both directions and know he has been cheated. "I feel like I was adopted," I complained to my father many years ago. "You were," he laughed. The old man always thought he was funnier than I did.

Meredith was banished to the early-morning news after Gabe's birth. I went to CNN to profile presidential candidates heading into 1992, then produced a CNN documentary on the Democratic nominee, Bill Clinton, with my pal Ken Bode, late of NBC News and PBS's *Washington Week in Review*. Lily Max, our daughter, arrived after the inauguration and took Meredith off the predawn hook. Soon after, she left CBS for good. Her instinctive sense of the value of family was reassuring. Every member of the family was a vital player, and the whole, the family itself, was greater than the sum of its parts.

Anyone battling chronic illness understands the power of family support and even the groundless fear of being left. Those of us who do battle with such sickness can come to think or fear that we drain our families emotionally, taking more than we give. Such fears are the psychological baggage we must carry. Too often, we are blind to the fact that even in our pain, we give to our loved ones, even as we receive.

It is almost instinctive by now. If there is a child around when I have a bad moment, unleashing my temper on myself in frustration, I try to redress the balance by engaging my young witness constructively on any subject that comes to mind. I need that kid to see my better side as quickly as possible.

When I slipped and fell from the bottom few steps in the foyer, "Damn it!" escaped from my lips spontaneously. I saw Lily around the corner in the living room ignoring me. This was business as usual for her, but I pulled her over to the piano to show her how to play "Für Elise," a Beethoven song she was struggling with. My hands do not work so well, but she got the gist. We were back on track.

I bounced around television for a year, sorting out my world and facing the hard fact that life's little tasks were getting larger and more difficult. My right leg had become so weak, I was unable to lift it. If I wanted to cross my right leg over my left as I sat, I had to lift it with my hands and place it over the other leg. On the street, that weakness meant falling in the gutter as my foot failed to clear a curb or tripping over sidewalk cracks and sprawling forward on my face. By the time I went to Fox in 1994 to run the public affairs component of a cable start-up, called *fx*, humiliating falls in the street were regular events.

It was not only my leg that was going numb. I could not lift my arm above my head to hail a cab. And my right hand had been neutralized. My writing was no longer legible. I signed checks with the initials for my first and middle names because it had become too difficult to write out my name in full. Brushing my teeth and shaving became arduous tasks. Combing my hair was an ordeal. There were regular determined decisions to grow a beard, thwarted only by the apparent fact that my appearance with three colors of facial hair was disconcerting. Ulysses S. Grant, it turned out, I was not.

I was beginning to view myself as a diminished person and holding myself accountable. Self-recrimination made no sense, but there it was, an emotional pattern I would fight forever. Most upsetting to me was that my children could see it all. I was moving into that phase where illness can no longer be hidden or explained away. I was wearing the scarlet letters *MS*. My guiding principle had long been, Do not lie and do not tell the truth too openly. That approach was quickly growing obsolete.

nine

No Secrets

The night I catapulted backward down the stairs, landing on my head in the foyer, there was a small audience that gasped and shrank away in horror. "Are you all right, Dad?" Ben cried tentatively from a safe distance. The kids were freaked. These young witnesses had taken in the event just before bedtime, and the family secret predictably and finally trickled out in small beds in the night.

"Mom, tell me. What is going on," was Ben's blunt demand. No more BS was his urgent message. Ben was not about to confront me. Upset was great and questions came in earnest. The kids were all under ten, and they were scared. For a long time, these children had known little enough about my physical problems, but they did understand something was amiss. My damaged vision was apparent to all, though handled so casually that bad eyesight just seemed to be a part of who I was. Ben laughed and told a friend once, "My dad can't see anything."

Still, nothing specific about MS had been said to them. Meredith and I felt strongly that they were entitled to a childhood that would be as carefree as we could choreograph. Still, they had begun picking up that more than vision was broken. My stumbles were frequent and obvious.

The night of the stairs became the moment that the whole truth was put on the table. Meredith told me later that she thought mystery only made reality more foreboding. "It was time to say something," she remembers. "The kids were flipped out." Meredith took on the task. The *M* word was spoken, multiple sclerosis being an unknown to these little ones. Naming the disease, she thought, would demystify events and accelerate the process of coming to grips with Daddy, an assignment these kids probably will never complete for many reasons.

Openness felt right. My children were old enough to deserve the truth. And truth took the pressure off us all. Closet illness serves no one. Flinging wide the doors allowed the

157

kids to grow comfortable with a physically flawed parent and proved to be healthy. My kids have learned the positive lesson that physical perfection is less important than tolerance and love. I will never be perfect, and neither will the kids, contrary to what their mom seems to believe. My children's sense of security does seem to come from our love and their knowledge that they will always know about important events in our house.

The openness at home signaled a change in attitude for me and inaugurated a slowly evolving public candor. At *fx*, the Fox cable start-up where I was an executive producer, the television studio floor was strewn with cables, snaking around the crowded space. I would trip over those rubber reptiles as I went about my business, unable to quite lift my right foot high enough. And I was falling on the avenues of New York. I was sick of television entertainment disguised as news, and my health was deteriorating. I wanted out from TV and MS. Only one was possible.

Twenty-five years after deciding that television news was my chosen career and mission, I left the business. Parting was neither sweet nor sorrowful. I had run out of places to hang my hat and was tired of seeking jobs

I did not want from people who did not want to hire me.

Bill Moyers had listened to my fury and frustrations many times over and had shaken his head, saying, "You can never leave the news business, Richard. For you, it is a calling." A calling. It was a wrong number. My messianic complex had run its course. The world would be saved without me.

My crumbling health, specifically my crumbling legs, led to another watershed decision. I decided I needed the help of a cane. A cane. The ultimate crutch. The decision was mine alone; no one told me to get a cane, no doctor announced that it was time. Common sense had just overtaken me. Too much time had been spent stumbling in streets, falling on stairs. My explosions of anger were growing boring. Just maintaining my equilibrium was a struggle. Finding relief could wait no longer.

I was walking across West Fifty-seventh Street on an errand one day, glancing at Carnegie Hall across the busy street and planning no life-changing events. Then I stopped in my tracks. I was standing directly in front of Uncle Sam's, a famous old cane and umbrella store (gone now). I stood staring at the large windows and just musing. Then I ducked through the door.

"This store has been here since Grant was president," the old proprietor told me. "Were you working here then?" I asked. The white-haired gentleman smiled and nodded. "What kind of umbrella are you looking for?" I was momentarily speechless. "I am looking for a cane," I said evenly. "A cane?" he asked. "Do you want to look as old as I am?" That will happen soon enough, I thought.

For a while after taking up a cane, I felt like an exhibitionist, parading my problems for all to see. My new wooden stick was in my mind a neon statement of vulnerability that villagers could see at great distances. After thirteen years of living with MS, I was throwing in the towel in my long war against admitting weakness.

My relief was complete, even compelling. The unspoken lie had evaporated. I was what I was, and it did not matter anymore. The honest explanation for a cane in my possession came easily. More important, my self-deception stopped because it was no longer possible. Denial had taken me far. Reality would carry me the rest of the way.

Only when cane was in hand did I realize what erroneous assumptions about me were loose in the land. My damaged equilibrium had convinced some that I was a garden-variety drunk. I swayed and staggered as if I were pouring whiskey sours on my cereal in the morning. That, coupled with the slight slur that overtakes my speech when I am tired, made me an inebriate to the world.

Once I was refused service in midafternoon at a liquor store as I tried to buy a bottle of wine to take home. "You are not feeling well," the clerk had said quietly. "You should go home." I was furious at the assumption. The police routinely had been following me up the hill from the train at the end of the day, presumably watching to see if I could stagger home in my drunken condition. And a neighbor, on seeing the cane for the first time at a soccer game, asked Meredith what was wrong with me. She was relieved by the answer. "Only MS? We thought he had a drinking problem," she admitted.

The cane did make me feel old, but it has become a constant companion, its value clearer with every step. The cane provides the third leg of my human tripod and is a source of significant support. Seven years have passed since we joined forces, and I will not leave home without it. The sleek, even chic, glossy instrument has become a piece of my identity. Whither I goest, the cane is sure to go. It is included in my comfortable snapshot of myself.

My cane led me haltingly to my epiphany. Finally I was understanding that progressive diseases progress. This was for real, probably forever. Changes in my body and the increased difficulty of functioning became impossible even for me to ignore. When nobody knew, illness did not exist. Living on the edge had worked for what seemed a long time, but that period was now over. Beirut to Beijing, Warsaw to Washington had dissolved to riding the number 1 subway down Broadway in the hope of making it from point A to point B without killing, stumbling, or otherwise embarrassing myself. The decision to ratchet back my demands on myself became a campaign to get real that, in the end, was unburdening.

The one secret that remained was just how difficult day-to-day life had become for me. There was no self-pity, but no point in sharing the details. For all my fumbling limbs, my experience with multiple sclerosis was centered in my eyes. Eyes, it has been written, are the window to the soul. Injure my eyes and you have bruised my very being. Here, too, patience is the first order of business. But coping with a significant loss of vision requires more than patience. Recalibrating all that is to be expected from life, a painful but necessary personal journey, must be undertaken. Other senses must be retrained, from ears to fingers to nose, Tinkers to Evers to Chance.

Life is eyesight intensive. I see that every day, though through an imperfect lens. The streets of New York hold special appeal in the early morning, when sunlight glances off buildings in the sky, and on the ground traffic builds and pedestrians start choking on exhaust fumes. Few are on the streets at this hour. Most shops were not even open one day as I headed for an early routine appointment with my lawyer. As I ambled down Seventh Avenue by Carnegie Hall and turned the corner, I saw a coffee shop and turned in for a bagel.

I realized I was standing in the kitchen, looking on as sweating men in white aprons worked the ovens. Glancing to my left, I saw the doorway to the dining room and headed toward the opening. As I approached, I saw a man heading into the same space from the opposite direction. I moved to my left to let him pass. He chose the same direction. I stepped to the right. The guy made the same move. This character obviously was one of those New Yorkers who delights in picking a fight. I looked up, my jaw rigid as my temper flashed. I was ready to at least tell off the jerk.

And there I was, trembling slightly, fist clenched, standing before a full-length mirror, dancing with myself and ready to do battle with a now familiar fellow wearing the jacket I had donned less than an hour earlier. The men at the ovens had paused to silently watch my performance. Their slack jaws revealed mute astonishment.

Writing about my travels above- and below-ground in this great city sounds like a complaint list. That it is not. Adventure is great, and this is just how my life goes. One cannot concentrate on coping without admitting what he is coping with. My kitchen choreography had opened and closed in one day. But the show goes on. The drama showcases the blunders that regularly travel with those with impaired vision.

For me, these mild mishaps momentarily marry my rage at my legal blindness and my laughter at these absurd events. Those of us with seriously flawed vision see our worlds in very eccentric ways. We view our lives through distorted lenses. Our emotional reactions vary, based on how foolish we assume we look and how vulnerable we feel at any given time.

Timidity and self-consciousness have been slowly overcome, replaced by today's casual nonchalance at walking into undesirable situations, not to mention a wall, and spending a lot of time lost. Just learning to ask for help or directions took work, but now the ability to do either has become an invaluable coping skill. The best is saved for underground.

In my early days of obscured vision, I restricted my journeys to bus rides. Slowly came the skill to survive the New York City subway system, a proving ground for the visually impaired. Every imaginable challenge, from personal safety to negotiating a trip to an unfamiliar destination, is there.

My regular forays into the subways become descents into an unsettling fog that envelops the vague forms of humanity in motion. The rumble and vibrations of thundering trains on the move add their punctuation. I struggle to stay on my feet and see where I am going. I have glanced off of poles, tripped and fallen up and down stairs. I often cannot read the numbers or letters on trains as they enter the station.

Every light down below screams "Caution." I use my other senses as a hidden guidance system. My ears tell me when a train is approaching, when there is an argument just up the platform. My nose says where to sit. Some subway riders also happen to live down there, sleeping on trains or behind wastebaskets, panhandling and parading their fumes, not the sweetest companions for an outing on the number 1 train.

The primary rule of the subway is: Do not make eye contact with anyone. It holds true even for people with impaired sight who have to stare intently to take in and make sense of the images of life. Ogling a woman can be mistaken for engagement or misunderstood as worse.

Aboveground, the circus continues. Walking in the city is running the gauntlet. I must watch my feet to see that I do not trip over sidewalk cracks. I watch for traffic because I move slowly in the street. Yet I may be the only legally blind jaywalker in the city. My radar is technically perfect, with ears that guide, helping me gauge speed by the sound of the engine. This is when eye contact counts. The hard stare at drivers is unflinching. I dare them to run me over. They always back down. So far. Finding addresses is no such sport. I crane and search, crossing streets back and forth, stumbling down curbs.

I get there. I just leave a little early. Traveling my world is a negotiation without end, an ongoing bargain with myself. To keep my cool is to honor the agreement. Living with disability requires quiet resolve. I know a calm patience I never possessed before. The ability to laugh at my comic missteps allows me to get where I am going and simultaneously provides entertainment in the streets.

My battle is to find a basic comfort level with the baggage I carry wherever I go. My condition is no secret. I have talked and written about my brushes with illness enough that I must forfeit any claims of privacy. Privacy belongs to those who feel they cannot reveal limitations they will not admit to themselves.

I admit them, and so does Meredith. When Meredith landed on *The View*, it quickly became clear that she was going to put her life on television. We discussed if and when candor should include my illness. "That is up to you," Meredith said with a shrug, "but talking about it would demystify the disease and maybe help others in the same boat." I hemmed and hawed and said to do it if she was so moved. And she has been, occasionally. With the enthusiasm of converts, we both get satisfaction from the

167

casual on-air acknowledgments of multiple sclerosis.

Over the seven seasons of *The View*, Meredith has gone far beyond MS when she talks about me, and frequently I have gotten burned. Meredith discovered a foil. Me. And she really was funny. I became her eccentric husband, not her suffering spouse. The more grief I take, the less I believe anyone could feel sorry for me.

"Richard would sleep with a ham sandwich," she says in her understated, casual tone to an audience of millions around the country. I would not, of course, though a steak sandwich might be nice. We were on the record about our problems and obviously ignoring them. That felt just right.

The single MS-related struggle that remained private and could not be ignored was what I understood the least about with my illness. By the mid-nineties, cognitive problems had become the most threatening, yet the quietest, of MS enemies. Outsiders see the canes and wheelchairs and can know many of the problems, but they cannot really understand the slow, secret pain of a mind that is slowly ceasing to work as it should.

There is nothing obvious to the outside world about that. Even our loved ones, those closest to us, find it difficult to identify the problems. Changes are slow, and they can be subtle. When my talking slows to the painful pace of groping for words, Meredith waves her hands toward me, thrown and threatened by this problem and trying to pull the words from me. Hurry up, she is saying. Please. "Relax," I tell her. "This is real life, not a television talk show."

I seek safe passage across the black holes, the dark and silent pockets of the mind. Where once there was the precision of specific words, information, or ideas, now there are halting silences. Vacuums. I cannot reach deeply enough into myself to pull them out intact or in time to make my point.

Small confusion leads to large frustration. What to do next about anything in any context used to amount to a routine if not remote control operation. Now such considerations can stop me cold, as if there is anything at stake. A former colleague used to tell me that he thought Emmett Kelly was my tailor. Fair enough. I am the worst-dressed person I know. Yet I cannot just get dressed efficiently anymore. I used to wear whatever I could find, and now I find that I cannot wear anything without a struggle in my head.

I place my reading glasses on the washing

machine as I move clothes out of the dryer. My eyes dart over to the washer a few times to remind myself that the glasses are there. When the clothes are in the basket, I begin the wild search for the glasses. Even for me, that is not normal. I ride the subway shuttle from Grand Central to Times Square to change subway lines and travel uptown. Instead I find myself on the street wondering why I am there.

Conceptualizing simple tasks is difficult. I sit on the train into New York in the morning, armed with a backpack, assorted books and papers, and, of course, my cane. When the train pulls into Grand Central and it is time to stand, quick decisions about which article to put in what hand drive me crazy. Frequently, something falls to the floor. This is happening because I am in my fifties, I reassure myself, though I do not believe that for a second. This feels different, way out of proportion to the challenge. Is this the price tag for too many good times in the 1960s? I think not.

Fifty percent of patients with multiple sclerosis experience difficulties with cognition, though when I am sitting at the computer, losing my train of thought and finding it suddenly impossible to make sense of any spelling of a simple enough word, it is only I who have this problem.

There is little one can do to find ways out of the darkness. When the kids go to their mother for help with homework, it is all too obvious why they walk around me. I can find simple instructions baffling. Soon the children are helping me. My frustration feeds their own.

Doing her homework, Lily has groaned as she's seen me coming. "I'm okay, Dad. Honest," my little girl insists, followed soon enough by the soft call to her mother. "Mom, I need you." My feelings of helplessness will not go away. Humiliation is sitting with a child who calls out to Mom in the next room for the answer to a question I could have provided easily. My cognitive crimes are punishable with the unintended insult followed by searing self-doubt. This is not my leg or foot or hand, but my mind.

The dreadful possibility of a limited mind brings a chilling fear that will not go away and a renewed determination to keep my sense of humor well lubricated. My accommodation with multiple sclerosis has otherwise come, though slowly, and I now see the illness as cohabiting intimately with me in my body. I've even come to believe that I might be a better, even gentler person for the baggage I must carry through life. The ride may be rough. It is exhilarating. Few get to play the high-stakes game and learn so much about themselves in the process. Boredom, not pain, is the enemy in life, and my life is not boring. Illness instructs.

My friends shake their heads when they hear me talk in this insistent upbeat way. It makes them crazy. They view my habit of drawing the positive from the pain as consummate madness. I tell them that if my afflictions were not so threatening, they might be worth having. I like to watch their faces when I say that. People who go through life without serious health problems are fortunate. I have a gift, though. Believe it. I cannot imagine a life without illness. But understand this. Said sentiment does not numb the raw nerve.

My advice to myself is simple. Run with MS, not away from it. That race from existing illness cannot be won. See the truth. We move forward with grace when the wind is at our backs.

If peace of mind had not come with the end of an awkward secret, at least there was no longer a state of war raging inside of me. I was surviving well enough, and surviving well is winning. There was something else out there, however. A second predator was lurking. What was hiding just around the corner would be devastating. People who suffer through a difficult illness often believe they are indemnified against further calamity. That assumption, as it turned out for me, could not have been further from the truth.

ten

Free Fall

"You do not want to hear this, I'm sure," the internist's practiced mantra began, "but you are over fifty, and you really should get a routine colonoscopy." Right. The advice was duly filed. Somewhere. I had spent too many years ignoring too much medical advice to get too worried. I had undergone too many hideous treatments to get exercised at the thought of an invasive procedure that I just might not get around to enjoying.

That night, I dreamed I was standing around a party in a glass house with clear walls between rooms. The gathering was under way, the house crowded and noisy. I was looking for my old colleague and friend Mark, an affable guy who had died a horrible death from cancer only months earlier. I felt a sense of urgency. I did not know why, though I knew he was searching for me, too. I milled around, gazing through walls until I spotted him. Our eyes met.

Mark looked as sick as I remembered, pale and gaunt, hairless from chemotherapy. He wore the red bandanna that he had sported at the end of his life. We shook hands and said nothing. Somehow, we did not need to speak. The dream ended. The next morning, feeling shaken, I gritted my teeth and made the appointment for the colonoscopy.

On a windy October day in 1999, the procedure was done. The first call came as I was in Houston, interviewing Dr. Michael DeBakey for a documentary about medical research. "I'm sure it is nothing," DeBakey said in his slow, soft drawl when I casually mentioned the call after our session. Something told me otherwise. "Your doctor probably wants to tell you the polyp he removed was benign."

Not quite. "The polyp was malignant," my internist announced when his call caught up with me in Washington in the next days. "We've been looking all over for you." That polyp in my colon, the one the doctor said was probably nothing, you know, no big thing, was malignant. Boom. Let the mind games begin. The dialectic of angst was unleashed and upon me. My all-purpose thesis, however rosy and ridiculous, had told me throughout my battles with MS that I am the captain, and my life will proceed as directed.

Now, along came a highly charged antithesis screaming, "Man the lifeboats." My power to steer my ship had been ruinously compromised by even rougher waters. I was being carried to a new place, unknown and unlike any other, and out of sight. That is what scared me most, not seeing the river ahead.

The struggle was for calm and composure. Meredith was calm, almost used to this brand of unhappy scenario. "You are not going to believe this," I had said when I called her from the New York train I immediately jumped in Washington. "Oh, I believe it," she replied quietly. "We can handle it." The next day, we were in the surgeon's office for an exam. Soon I went under the knife, the surgeon removing my coccyx and going through my lower back. "Access to the middle portion of the rectum is greater from that angle," he told me later. I hurt for months.

The surgery resulted in considerable post-op pain and also caused so much stress on my body that it jump-started the multiple sclerosis. Cancer and MS are not buddies. I had difficulty walking and using my right hand. I wound up shaving with my left hand, easy enough. Not so brushing my teeth. At a follow-up exam a few months later, a Sloan-Kettering oncologist told me to go home, that no further treatment was necessary, "You are too healthy to be here," he said, smiling. "Go." I did not need to hear that twice. Recognizing good fortune when it was thrust in my face, I stumbled down the stairs to the subway, feeling that I had cheated death.

As I left the hospital, I ran into Dan Rather's old secretary, later a producer on *West 57th*. "What are you doing here?" I asked. Tears welled in her eyes. "I have stage-three colon cancer." She grabbed my arm and turned toward the elevator. I was lucky. They had caught the cancer early, and I was safe.

In October, I went in for a repeat of the colon cancer screening. The colonoscopy now seemed routine. When I arrived at my office the following Monday, a chilling message to call the gastroenterologist was waiting. That was the entire message. Just call. I sat, silently looking at the phone for a while. I was certain that the news would be bad. I had come so far, managing MS and beating cancer. It was apparent, now, that I had not won. Calmly, I told myself I would do what I had to again. I marveled at my own inner strength. We are much tougher than we think.

The cancer indeed had come roaring back, to the site where the surgeon had gone, cutting out the first malignancy and calling me cancer-free. This turn of events was hard to believe and almost impossible to put into perspective. I had not made it a full year. I just sat, feeling paralyzed and staring out at the river. A barge was struggling up the Hudson. I always seem to be moving against the current, I thought.

A decision about how to react for the long haul came soon enough. To me, there is only one response — to seek personal strength and determination. But the initial thought process is not necessarily thoughtful. The impulse is almost knee-jerk, a gut reaction. Whatever the final product of this process, I have discovered, it rules the mind for the duration of the disease, speaking on a very basic level to who an individual is as a person.

A voice deep inside told me to toe the line, to remain calm and go for it. There was no bravery here, no posturing, only me taking the path of least resistance. It was a solitary moment. I felt numb but intended to survive. Shouting in anger was pointless; moaning and groaning a waste of time. Life is not fair. There is no one to sue.

Surgery this time would be aggressive. Invasive. My rectum, the site of the cancer and bottom of the colon, would be cut out, replaced by intestine pulled down from above. A bag, The Bag, might be necessary, joining my body at least temporarily to allow stitches to heal. There were a thousand questions on my lips and little certainty.

In the weeks before surgery there was work to do, with my family and in my own head. The thunderclaps kept coming. "The CT scan shows a spot on your liver." Boom. Lightning. This was not the opening remark one expects from the surgeon preparing me, I thought, for something quite different. I already was facing colon cancer, now the man in green was talking about possible liver cancer. Whatever else the surgeon said was lost to me. My heart shared shoes with my feet, and the clamor in my head was deafening. I felt the shivering presence of my mortality in the chilly examining room on that gray November day.

The pursuit of calm was under way one more time. This was a period of intense self-absorption. But recognizing the needs of others, small people in particular, had to go to the front of the line. Thinking of my children made it easier to think of myself. Because it offered perspective. We are a family, and this was one big and messy package. The need now was to maintain my equilibrium, to locate my wits and keep them as close as I hold my kids.

One cannot fight in a prone position. Stand up, I told myself. Too many people try fighting while flat on their backs, just flailing away like a fish out of water. Individuals can panic and underestimate their own fortitude. Individuals in pain are unable to see their emotional strength, unable even to see the blue of the sky. I chose to embrace the cancer. It was part of me now. Why take chances by making it angry? I wanted to understand the disease. Charm the beast. "Keep your friends close," the Godfather instructed, "and your enemies closer."

Cancer was the enemy at the gate, the surgeon my commander in chief. The spot on my liver was probably nothing, he told me, the mark perhaps of an old athletic injury or a benign cyst. "These scans show everything, every dent in the fender," the radiologist explained. I was not mollified.

But I did not panic, either because I had the presence of mind to adopt a wait-and-see attitude or because I had pitched forward into a steeper denial than I had ever experienced with MS. Either way, I knew the truth would be knocking at the locked door soon enough.

Knowing a lot has always been important to me. And again I knew nothing. The lack of knowledge felt dangerous because emotion might fill the void. At the moment, emotion felt like nothing to mess with. An information vacuum offers a hiding place and provides scant fuel to proceed toward panic.

I did have the distinct sense that there was no malignancy in my liver. The blood studies were normal. I had none of the likely side effects of liver cancer. I had not done anything wrong. Nobody was particularly angry with me. And I did not deserve to die. The logic was peculiar, but my case was airtight.

"Let's be sure here. I want you to get a PET scan," the surgeon said. It sounded like a machine the vet throws dogs into from time to time. One hair-raising visit to the dark subbasement of the hospital, with its imposing high-tech machines whirring and quietly invading the internal privacy of the prostrate patients, would resolve the mystery. PET stands for positron emission tomography, the ultimate in high-tech medicine. A PET scan uses radioactive glucose to highlight any malignancies in the body.

My postdawn trek to the hospital from the train included a detour around Harlem's Marcus Garvey Park on Upper Fifth Avenue. The walk was calming, the folks on the street charming. Smiles were reassuring. I arrived at the hospital early and nervously looked around. Strange technicians in white coats greeted me. I walked down a corridor and looked into open rooms where a myriad of legs protruded from machines. They appeared dead.

The IV glucose drip began to circulate through my body as I was placed on a short conveyor belt and thrust into a metal tunnel with a second-by-second digital readout. I was convinced that when the meter hit zero I would be launched through the ceiling and into space. A Mozart piano concerto played in perfect stereo behind me. Hushed voices speaking technical gibberish were audible, though not understandable. This was space-age medicine and completely alienating. I yearned for something homier. A simple sofa would suffice.

The procedure ended as quietly as it began. I just lay there, wondering what was next. I was excused and told to dress. After ten or fifteen minutes, a resident approached me, asking if I used a cane. "What about my liver?" I inquired less than gently. The guy ignored me. "You have stress in your left shoulder, a hot spot, probably from the constant use of the cane in your left hand," he went on. "Right?" Are you out of your mind? I screamed in my head. "Your liver is clean," the young robot finally added, almost as an afterthought.

My colon cancer remained, but I felt curiously safe at that moment. The crisis had passed because the death sentence had been lifted. I still had MS and cancer, but I felt a new confidence that I would prevail. Bad situations call for perspective.

The prospect of liver cancer, however remote, had brought my second duel with colon cancer into sharper focus. All around me were very sick people. Cancer was spread up and down the halls, I imagined. My gaze traveled beyond my own body to see the suffering of others around me. I was transfixed. By taking stock of the suffering of others, horrifying myself over and over with their imaginable pain, my own was muted. These case studies at a distance seemed deeply rooted in my own need to endlessly evaluate the relative severity of my own suffering. I went to my surgery believing that others faced ordeals far worse than mine. This was oddly comforting.

The fog was lifting as I sluggishly awoke after almost seven hours of surgery and the day's deep sleep. Anesthesia imposes nothingness, with no sense of events or the passage of time. Suddenly, there is consciousness. And a breathing tube down my throat. And pain. The tube would come out only when the doctors were convinced that MS would not rob me of breath. An anesthesiologist hovered, hurriedly showing me how to administer morphine every five minutes or so. Everyone was in a hurry, including me. I wanted just one answer and did not ask my good wife if I was going to live or die. My interest in those small matters depended on the other answer I immediately demanded.

"The bag," I whispered. "Do I have a bag?" I asked. "Yes. You do," Meredith replied softly. "I'm so sorry." Meredith noted later that I was immediately crestfallen. "You have an ileostomy, and it is temporary. Really." God, the bag. This was no goody bag. What next? My self-indulgent horror of the bag was primal. I suspect I am not alone in that regard.

To hell with the cancer, I screamed silently. Now I had bigger fish to fry, eat, and digest. The ileostomy presented a quality-of-life issue that absorbed my fears. Trivializing the *Big C* seemed to be what I was doing as I veered off course and focused on this sideshow in the rollicking cancer circus. Sidetracking anxiety to the point of absurdity was a detour for my emotions. I was horrified by the tube of flesh protruding from my belly, my pipeline to the bag.

I avoided the mirror in the bathroom, even keeping the medicine cabinet open to avoid the quick, accidental glance at my body. I stood at the sink, naked, just staring when I returned from the hospital. All I saw was this bag, outlined in blinking neon red. I felt diminished, even emasculated. "Richard, are you going to stop standing there?" Meredith would ask. "You look exactly the way you did yesterday."

There were the mishaps, the bag that broke, the one with the leak. The day the bag just fell off during a business lunch as I sat quietly at a diner was so embarrassing that I started to laugh. "I have to go now," I said calmly. "My bag broke. You know how annoying that can be." Mostly, I learned to be careful and conservative and to take no chances. Misadventures seemed to go curiously undetected. The big hurdle seemed to be the very idea of the bag.

A man should not be hanging this purse at his waist, I thought. A rabbit pelt dangling from a coarse old rope, perhaps. The old pouch should be made of stained leather and hang next to his hunting knife, just over the notches in his belt, which, of course, should be many. A sissy pouch for transporting that to which every manly man turns a blind eye was not acceptable. Never, I thought defiantly.

The scene was silly, pointing up the need to choose battles carefully in a long fight. And I maintained a quiet though steady level of private embarrassment at my wimpy attitude. I was a cancer survivor, a member of that elite club to which every cancer victim surely applies. A temporary ileostomy was the least of my worries, a small price to pay for life. I laughed ruefully, bitterly, at the situation and at myself. I knew I was acting out in my head like a child, but I could not stop myself.

My gyroscope was broken. I was off-kilter, looking at my life from the wrong angle. The fact that I was now cancer-free should have made me feel relieved and grateful, but it was lost on a churning mind.

Life on the bag was temporary — just a three-month sentence — yet to accept it and adjust would have felt like giving in.

My obsession was about seizing whatever small control I still had over my body. MS had seized significant control long ago. This was icing on the cake. I was in the hands of a doctor I barely knew, fighting a disease I knew nothing about except that it was a mortal enemy. It was that unambiguous erosion of the ability to control my life, to guard and guide my health, that so threatened me. This new disease was a sly, well-armed adversary. The cancer was stealthy and strong, dangerous, if not deadly, even for the fit.

I felt totally vulnerable.

My return from the hospital had collided with other bad news, word of my friend Helene's death. Her encouraging words had sent me off to battle my cancer. Now she was dead of her own. I had watched and listened as Helene was slowly slipping away. The last leg of her journey had taught poignant lessons for continuing mine. As Helene's life was ebbing, her grace in the face of a certain end was striking. She would tell me that this was not a question of what but when. Her challenge was to figure out how to finish the journey in peace. Her young daughters were her life, and they were her focus.

For a brief moment I realized how lucky I was. Coping with a hard life is vastly preferable to dealing with certain death. Helene had spoken of what she had learned about herself throughout her ordeal. She told me she had given too much of herself to her law firm and not enough to her kids. I doubt that. Helene would smile and tell me that she finally noticed beauty around her, that she now appreciated flowers and skies and smells. "It took me a long time to learn to cope with what is happening," she said.

Events in my life kept playing out. Pain dissipated. The ileostomy went, reversed as promised after three months. But things went terribly wrong very quickly. My plumbing could not be restored. The pain and shame that followed were extraordinary. Every device for remaining calm and upbeat was challenged. I was plunged into a despair I had never known.

The beast was in there. I knew it. I could feel the creature writhing in my belly, in my waking hours and throughout the dark night when I swore I could hear the snarling.

And the stuff just poured out of me, moving with the relentless flow of lava that cannot be halted. Poop, my kids used to call it, before discovering more colorful language. More than fifty years had passed in my life, and I was traveling that all too inevitable full circle back to infancy and painful feelings of humiliation that came well ahead of their time.

People do not outgrow the shame of their bowels. Even as adults, we have demons in our gut. Mine was a monster, angry and trapped, pushing everything out of its way to escape. "There is shit everywhere," Kurt Vonnegut wrote of his weariness almost thirty years ago, telling the story of his wife's tortured death from cancer in the preface to *Welcome to the Monkey House*, a collection of short stories. Nothing has changed. Vonnegut's memory of "shit everywhere" and the murmurings of "no pain" were what he remembered of his wife's grim demise.

I held my belly constantly and sometimes doubled over with waves of intense cramps. The psychic duress was searing. My life and everything around me was a mess. Productivity stopped. It was hard to think of anything above my waist.

Despair overtook me. That darkness washed over my body but did not clean it. The surgeon explained that the rectum, the south end of the colon, was probably closing at a point three or four inches in. He said the stricture undoubtedly was causing the pain and control problems. The doctor added that no sphincter muscles on the planet, even in a healthy person, could hold forth under such conditions. A surgical solution was possible. Hope replaced despair.

My next surgery occurred on a late May morning in 2001. It felt like March. It was cold, and the rain traveled sideways as Meredith and I left for the hospital before dawn. "Meredith," the nurse's aide called out when we arrived. "Hey, honey," an orderly yelled from down the hall. "What are you doing here?" "Dumping him," Meredith answered, pointing at me and smiling.

The operation immediately ended the problem. This had been the worst ordeal I ever encountered, but the agony did seem to end. My private tour of hell called into question every coping device I thought I owned. I had let loose my fear and depression, and they had run amok. I became as dark as what seemed to be enveloping me. "Coping, I ain't," I kept saying to Meredith. "Coping, you is," she would answer charitably.

Coping shines brightest when it comes easy. Living and functioning with multiple sclerosis had become routine. Thirty years of adjusting and compromising with my body were second nature. Calmly negotiating my world, as if by remote control, was my life.

The surgeon had reopened my colon, but five days later it shut down again and I was consumed by an overwhelming anger. Standing at the base of the stairs, I would scream with rage, "I can't take this." "Richard, please don't do this," Meredith would plead. "There are children in the house." "So what," came my answer. "They might as well know." I was unable to legislate words from the north end with the south end so out of control.

My anger scared me.

By now, my clothes were changed a half dozen times a day. The shrapnel from my bitter unhappiness struck everyone in sight. "I am not going to live here much longer," became an all-too-frequent refrain. Rage had seized me, and I was spewing. Where my children were when these eruptions came was of no concern. They were probably hiding.

"No," I went on. "I cannot live this way." My desperation filled the house. "I am out of here." Meredith believed I was threatening suicide. She took it seriously. I knew I was yelling about moving out of our home because I could not bear for my children to see me this way. My pain had been spread evenly in the family.

Neither depression nor suicide goes with my psyche. In fact, I have never had a suicidal moment in my life. My inner strength was cracking, though, and I was failing to distinguish between the permanent condition and a disruption that was temporary, albeit horrific. Again I needed perspective.

Perspective came in a wheelchair resting motionless. In it sat a man with no tone to his body and a head that fell forward. Here slumped a man whose health was tortured, a state that would last until death. I needed to horrify myself. I had to see, close up and with my own flawed eyes, a man who had descended into Hell. This human being did not have cancer, but multiple sclerosis.

For me, Larry was an example of the horrific possibilities of catastrophic illness. He was no stranger to thoughts of suicide. I had known of the man for a long time, although we never had met. I had wanted him not to exist. Now I needed him. I walked slowly up the hill to see him, to shock sense into myself in the midst of my pain.

The wheelchair carrying Larry went nowhere. He was an inmate. With great discomfort, I climbed the hill to meet him. "My life is torture," Larry told me without discernible emotion. "I am locked up in this body."

Larry was everything I feared that someday I would become. This was the man who had put the ABC News magazine *20/20* on the air as director of operations more than two decades ago. Now he did not often leave his bed. He sat in his wheelchair like stone, not able to move a muscle. He could not turn his head even slightly to attempt making eye contact. His arms and legs rested in precisely the same position for our entire visit. Not a finger moved. It could not.

"I don't go outside anymore," he said. "I don't want people to see me with my head hanging down because I cannot lift my chin." Larry's wife, Harriet, was almost always with him. Their son is not. He is grown and gone, and the nest seems very empty. "I think he needed to go far away," Harriet said later.

How do suffering people do it, I wondered. Larry's emotional pain was deeper than my own. What bubbling source of emotional sustenance becomes the deep reservoir of strength, I wondered. What sustains a suffering person? There is no answer. "I do not know what keeps me going," he says. "You just do it. Maybe it is for your wife, your child. Maybe it is because you do not know what else to do."

There needs to be a Plan B in my own life. I did not need the colon crisis to figure that out; cancer had only added urgency to the thought process. I have known that MS could be taking me to places I do not wish to spend the rest of my days. There are no round-trips offered. In midnight musings I have long believed that I might need a ticket out, up and away from the pain. Maybe not. Hopefully not. Certainly the time is not here. It may never come. I do not even know when or where the point of departure rests. I want to be ready, though.

"I think of suicide a lot," Larry told me. "Don't you? When I was driving and still going to work I had a tree picked out. I could have gotten that sucker up to eighty and hit that tree, and I would not have to go through this bullshit." Whether these options are fantasy or a function of good planning, they seem constructive enough. Suicide is control. Empowerment.

There is no happy resolution and, for some, no happy life. "You can either request permission to give up, which seems an awful thing to ask your wife and child, or you can participate in an awful big lie and commit suicide," Larry said to me.

"That is not fair either."

Larry told me he had a friend ready to assist when this man who could not move was ready to move on. Larry said that if and when the time came, he would go peacefully. When word spread through the community that Larry had died suddenly, I could only wonder.

People such as I draw strength from a person like Larry. Things could be worse, I say over and over, again and again, and to no one in particular. There is power to that point. The life far harder than mine has true meaning in evaluating my own journey. On a sparkling early autumn day, under a clear sky and a solid wood roof, a man and his wife were gracious hosts in their comfortable prison on the side of a quiet hill. They had gone on with their lives because at that moment they could see no options. What came later may never be known.

The strength to get by, I realized, is understated and powerful. We all do what we must as we try to make our lives work. Work, it is. Coping is quiet. There is no fanfare, no confetti. There are no parades. Just a quiet task aimed at emotional well-being, if not survival, pursued in subdued and sober tones and spoken in whispers, not shouts. The formula for successful coping rests in the eye of the beholder. There is no magic. We simply know it when we live it. Making peace is not a one-shot deal but an effort that spans a lifetime.

Coping takes discipline and self-control. They have long been my Holy Grail, the objects of a personal crusade. The quest for the quiet, reasoned responses had paid dividends. For me, there is a flip side to that coin, however: the temptation to move toward self-absorption. My pride in coping well had become an end, not a means. The house of cards tumbled easily when forcefully challenged.

An individual with illness is not the only person in pain. I lost sight of that fact. What I had to keep learning, observing myself in a crisis, with my family around me, my children in particular, is that the hurt and the fear spread outward in hard times. My coping had been selfish, centered on myself alone. Me. ME. *ME, ME, ME.* Me was all I could see.

That's the exact opposite of my old man. He stayed alone in his pain. And sometimes I felt just like the old man, in self-imposed exile, frequently just sitting and staring out any window, fixing on any tree or animal in the yard.

In the turmoil of cancer's complications,

my need to withdraw from all human contact, even in the family I loved, was real. I wanted to crawl under my own skin and hide. My habit of isolating myself was intense. That dynamic only magnified the loneliness of illness for me and the disturbing identity of outcast.

I learned the hard way that people are never in that crucible alone. Family and friends and close colleagues rub up against the despair we feel, but too frequently we do not raise our heads enough to see past ourselves.

For me, turning inward after cancer came shut out the light. I literally sat in dark rooms. Life became darker and darker. Darkness fed on itself. Perspective suffered. I learned that it takes time and a conscious effort to talk to those we love, to share fear and frustration without feeling weak.

Going it alone had been my badge of honor. How foolish. I confused silence with strength. I have come to see that as the classic male mistake. Shutting out others is weak and grossly unfair to those around us.

With my colon now shut down once more, I was now hostage to the medical establishment, practically taking up residence in offices around the city. I had been in the operating room so often, I asked the surgeon for a time-share. I was funny. And very angry.

We even tried dilating my rectum in the surgeon's office, without sedation. When I dropped off the ceiling, we decided "no more." Frustration finally drove me to a plan. I would take matters into my own hands. I persuaded the gastroenterologist, the colonoscopy king, to sedate me, dilate my rectum, and I would take it from there. I obtained the proper instruments from a medical supply house and learned to do the deed myself. The rectum would be fully dilated. Every day, for many months, I would arise at 4:45 a.m. and do what had to be done. The cat was my only witness. The self-taught, self-inflicted procedure worked.

And control of my body was mine once more. A powerful lesson had not been lost in the predawn darkness. The plan had been mine. I had pushed the guys in green out of the driver's seat and seized control of the car. I had hijacked my body, taken it back, if just for the moment. The gastroenterologist had liked the idea, the surgeon signing on a bit reluctantly.

I was taking personal responsibility, and that felt great. The procedure was unpleasant to be sure and no way to start the day. But taking charge was empowering. In a small way, even if just for those moments, the balance of power had shifted. A trying time now seemed to end, but the price was high.

"It tested everyone in this house," Meredith remembers. "You were tough, miserable, actually. A lot was inflicted on us, but we all did okay." Cancer seemed to cross the family wiring and cause a disconnect. The house had needed a giant sign, reading TILT. My frayed connection with my family weighed heavily on everyone, especially Meredith. The hospital had become her home, too. She stayed by my bed. My return to our other home became another ordeal. Everyone was at risk.

My cumulative, pent-up anger at illnesses had exploded, driving a wedge deep into our various relationships. The ordeal was hardest on Meredith. "I felt great distance from you after you came home from all that surgery," Meredith admits. "I would be lying if I did not tell you that I felt put off." I do not need to be told. I let go too much bile too often and still have not found my way home completely. "Your anger drove us all away."

Cancer in my life may be here to stay,

joining multiple sclerosis as the guest who will not leave. Though I am free of the actual cancer, the complications live on with no indication of tiring of their new home. Even the worst of the problems visit occasionally, as if to just let me know not to grow complacent. That message is heard loud and clear.

Cancer's most insidious complication had been anger. High emotion was born of pain and shame and fear, coming to visit in a time of crisis. Anger has yet to totally vacate the premises.

The love between children and parents may, in fact, be unqualified, but my children's bond with me was tested. The strains could not be hidden. We were surviving family madness from multiple sclerosis. That is tough enough. Cancer would place me almost out of reach.

eleven

The Kids
and Me

The morning the pancake fell to the floor and I hit the ceiling, the spatula was launched toward the wall, glancing off the kitchen window and into the sink. That shot heard round the house demonstrated once again that my anger can fly out of control at petty annoyances. The bellowing that accompanied the action betrayed my rage to everyone in the house unfortunate enough to miss the event. Anger is a staple in our kitchen, though I try to keep it out of sight, up in the cabinet, next to the flour.

Decades of battling multiple sclerosis have failed to produce the fail-safe system to short-circuit flashes of high emotion. I am not a perfect person. Failing eyesight, flawed hands, and a weak right arm had conspired to sabotage that pancake on this

Saturday morning. At least the dog was pleased. Combustion had been spontaneous, and, of course, I felt foolish.

Anger is my unyielding, live-in companion, though I have tried to break up that relationship for years. I alternate between fighting the flames and needing the heat. Losing my temper is the trigger for letting off steam, which builds all too fast. Chronic illness fuels the pressure cooker because the heat is turned up so regularly. My emotional hurt can find no resolution, and there is no release otherwise. Anger becomes the polar opposite of denial, an instant contradiction and the tacit, though highly charged, admission that the situation really does suck. Release brings relief, but too often with it comes humiliation. That is the price for my orgasms of anger. The fury feels good, then bad, and then I lose interest.

The kids try to ignore the occasional eruptions. There is enough noise in our family on any given day to go around. There are the predictable battles of three kids sharing two parents and the one objective of disrupting the peace whenever possible. As my health problems grew more intense, family tension has ratcheted up a level or two.

The kids are used to my temper. They are

not targets. The real target of the outburst remains the same. Me. They seem to understand that, though occasionally they have been struck by friendly fire. Their eyes are wide open, and they see the link between my physical flaws and frustration that boils over without warning. Their lives have been made more difficult by pressure born of wondering when Dad will go off next.

Illness is built into our lives. Sometimes it seems that illness is our lives. Our children see and understand. Their expectations of me are recalibrated when necessary and integrated into the game plan. Problems are not predictable, incidents can be ordinary or more dramatic than I would like. My fear is that anger will hurt my children and drive a wedge between us. That would kill me. I do think my kids have grown tough because they, too, are survivors. They see it all. Nobody could promise them a free ride.

Gabriel and I were alone in the house, abandoned by a busy family to fend for ourselves on a withering July evening. We headed out for an early supper at a local restaurant, ambling down a wide path known as the Aqueduct. Gabe and I were walking through the trees, enjoying the wildlife next to the Hudson River, and talking about his favorite baseball team, the Mets.

As Gabe ran ahead, I realized that I was having trouble with the heat, sweating profusely and finding it increasingly difficult to put one foot in front of the other and move forward. Anyone suffering from multiple sclerosis hears warning bells sound when heat is overpowering and legs begin to grow weak. A voice inside did warn me to turn back, that trouble lay ahead.

By now Gabe had run almost to town, and, anyway, I did not want to disappoint him. He wanted his usual favorite dish, chicken wings, and there was little food of any kind in our house. I shuffled along, growing angry and literally dragging myself down the hill and into the restaurant. I hoped no one would notice my difficulty or my growing edge. Gabe was focused on food and noticed nothing. An hour later we left, walking slowly across the street.

When I collapsed in the gutter on the other side of the road, the fall came without warning. My legs simply gave out. So did the happy grin on Gabe's face, which froze. There was no strength left for me to stand back up. My legs would not support me. Gabriel shrank into the entryway of a closed store as passersby and a waitress who had been watching from the restaurant rushed over to help. The anger rushed from me like air from a punctured tire.

My stinging pain came from watching Gabe, looking intently into his face as he turned away to avoid my gaze. The scene was haunting and the last thing I wanted my nine-year-old son to witness. His pain was apparent, the humiliation of this parent roaring in silently as I went down in slow motion. The apologies to all around me were self-conscious. This is my fault, I always think. This was unforgivable, as if there were a choice, because Gabe had walked and talked and laughed with me and now, once again, the poor kid was so vulnerable.

What goes through the mind of a child such as Gabe in a situation such as this is unimaginable. Here is a youngster, an athlete, for whom grace and physical perfection seem such an ideal. Gabe and his siblings see my stumblings and ignore my clumsiness, overlooking the profound limitations on my life and seeing whatever it is that can replace a fiercely protected ideal in their heads.

When I fall in a public place in their presence, with the added embarrassment of strangers present and eager to assist, my sickness is no longer the private issue of a family attempting to cope. The hurt in the faces of the children is clear and cannot be ignored or repainted by intense wishful thinking that life is fine.

My emotional apology to Gabe on this night was brushed aside by a child whose only wish seemed to be getting past what he had seen happen to his father. "That's okay, Dad," Gabe mumbled without emotion. "I know you couldn't help it." Gabe had seen this kind of theater performed to various audiences before. All my children have been there. The kids watch me like a hawk. They seem to chart every bad move and misstep. I constantly wonder if they see their futures in my failing body.

"Dad," Ben began to ask haltingly some years ago, "you know what is wrong with Grandpa?" The question came from nowhere. "Yes," I answered softly. "Is that what's wrong with you?" My heart skipped a beat. "It is, Ben." It was young Benjamin's turn to pause. "Is that going to happen to me?" The question pierced my armor. The inquiry was sobering. I thought for an hour in a moment and spoke slowly. "I do not know, Ben," I almost whispered, adding, "I hope not."

"I am going to get MS," Gabe announced on another day a few years ago. "You were a middle child, and so am I." The almost casual statement came devoid of obvious context. Something he saw in me at some arbitrary moment must have triggered the vulnerability he felt about himself. "I'll be okay," he assured me. "Don't worry."

There was no reassuring reply I could offer to any child of mine when a question about the future was raised. I could not bring myself to utter the predictable untruth, masquerading as the honest answer he or she sought. Perhaps reassurance was more important than truth. I did not know and had little time to ponder the question. The fact is, there is no certainty, and there can be no comforting answer to that haunting question.

When a genetic counselor told us in a routine conference before Ben's birth that genetic considerations did not exist with multiple sclerosis, we took her word at face value. Today, no counselor would give that assurance. If Meredith had questions or doubts, they went unasked, unanswered. My radar screen was shut off. Ben would be born within a month, and this seemed like the wrong time to ask questions for which there are no good answers. There continues to be no resolution to anxiety. Our history of miscarriages had turned our focus to just delivering a child. Sight beyond the day of birth was not in our minds. Three generations of MS in my family were gently put aside. Now the questions have grown large.

For thirty years, what lay down the road was a mystery. My life has changed, and I will always regret that the kids never saw me as what I was. I am less of a person than I used to be. My children never had the opportunity to see their father as the athlete, sweaty and strong and eager to take on all comers. The soccer player, the runner, are now the guy with the cane.

To the kids, I am only a spectator at their contests. Dad is there for them but always on the sidelines or in the stands. Kids know the score. They are the smartest people in the house, with keen eyes and powerful intuitive powers. The truth about sickness cannot be kept from kids, at least, not from my children. These not-so-little people need to see and understand and know. They must learn about illness and grow comfortable, becoming part of one family's determination to adapt.

A child's laughter goes a long way toward maintaining perspective about the future and identifying what is important in the life of a family. Kids define a family's culture, steering the coping process without true knowledge of the journey being undertaken.

Their influence is almost mystical. This is a truth about any family on this earth, though, of course, I see mine as special.

Meredith and I have our hands full. Our children are junior partners in the family corporation. We manufacture trouble. Each thinks he or she is chairman of the board and fights hard to ensure that no sibling, no puny partner seated across the table, is accruing too much family stock, in Mom's eyes especially.

Fifteen-year-old Ben is the titular head of the kid clan, or so he assumes. Ben plays the role of despot, occasionally the benevolent dictator, though I believe him to be a pretender. He has too much heart for that, and he seems to be kind to others outside the home, revealing a side he would never display for us. Ben is just the self-appointed fox guarding the chicken coop. What he says goes, but not too far. Ben is athletic and blond. We all know where those features will take a kid in our culture today. Ben is smart and savvy. He sees every trip, stumble, and fall. Ben feels my pain, a source of deep regret for me. I can do nothing to lift this emotional weight. In his own way, Ben understands the many dimensions of illness.

What Ben does not seem to understand

and makes no effort to is why his younger brother is allowed to walk the earth. When Gabriel was born, his two-year-old elder statesman brother paraded around a playroom thrusting his arms forward and saying "no" in steely tones, over and over. More than a decade later, Ben has not changed his mind.

Unlike his older brother, twelve-year-old Gabe is laid back and does not think he owns the world. Gabe has always demonstrated an unusual sensitivity toward others. This young man does not seek approval: in fact, he does not even care what others think. Gabe seems only to care about playing Nintendo. The second son plays to no audience but himself.

Gabe sets his own compass and listens to a voice in his head. What that voice tells him is a mystery. Gabe spares no sensibility in speaking his mind and asking the blunt questions others tiptoe around. Frequently, Gabe takes in the family drama and offers no reviews.

Lily Max, the little one, is the tough cookie. She is serious and disciplined, and she takes no prisoners. Lily fights off predators, brothers in particular, whom she scares with a snarl. My beautiful eleven-year-old daughter is a flower with sharp teeth. When it comes to living with brothers, Lily is a survivor.

Surviving the emotional rigors of dealing with Dad's declining health plays out across a childhood for a kid. Simply surviving is another matter. With physical limitations can come the inability to care for a child in an uncontrolled situation. I am haunted by my own frailties, my inability to protect a child of mine in a moment of need. That happened in 1992, when I almost killed Ben as we waited to catch a train. The incident took place in an instant.

Ben tumbled into the narrow space between train and platform like a shiny penny disappearing into his new ceramic piggybank. It was a slow-motion fall, a movie sequence that took but a moment. I was powerless to stop it. A quick glance up at me, devoid of all expression, and my boy vanished. The grown-up caution that guides the movements of a little boy, not yet four, had broken down, colliding with the loss of coordination that comes from my neurological illness.

We had held hands on the platform at that station because of the dangerous, wide gap between platform and train. The physical contact had felt good on this day. Ben needs me, too, I thought when he reached for me. I am so acutely aware of his magnetic link to his mother. We jumped onto the train, and then, as others came and went, walking on and off, Ben suddenly looked back at the platform and yelped, "Look, Dad. Your CNN card."

My work ID was lying on the platform by the open door. It surprised me, and I quickly told Ben to stay where he was while I fetched it. In an instant I was on the platform, only a long step from the doors, bent over and recovering my card. When I heard Ben yell, "Let me help," my hand shot up instinctively in the universal language of no.

The accident is a blur now, but I know I did it. I didn't know he had jumped to follow, and I think it was my extended arm that knocked him back and down the slot into the toaster. It took a moment to register that Ben was down. Squeezed in between platform and train, thousands of tons of huffing, wheezing steel, vibrating in anticipation and ready to roar on. No longer benign, this train was a metal monster about to eat my son.

I rescued Ben that morning, as surely as I had pushed him into danger and caused the crisis myself. My movements had been awkward, my equilibrium unsure. I had tried to react decisively, but my judgment was off. I could not see and chose the wrong action. Parent had failed child. I was not a fit guardian for a little one in that situation at that instant. Yet it was only a routine moment gone bad. Not to be there at all would have been to throw in the towel on my life and to rob a boy of an adventure with his father. I yelled to passengers to block the door so that the train would not move. I fell to my knees and reached down as far as I could, hanging down to the tracks and lifting a stunned child back to the platform.

The shiver of fear in my body has not gone away. For Ben, the memory of the awful incident has. A decade later, I do not travel anywhere in the city with a youngster in tow without replaying the videotape of that moment. My limitations are stored in the front of my mind. My movements are slow and deliberate, thought through and correct. There is, I discovered, no margin of error. Unintended consequences today are anticipated. This is what I must live with, the nightmare scenarios I confront every day.

There is the unintended consequence and the unforeseen event. When cancer came calling, explosives were thrown into the home of my children. Nobody was hit in the first attack. Meredith and I quickly agreed to tell the kids everything and answer all questions as honestly as we could. We sat them down and told the truth. Questions did come, first from Gabriel. "Are you going to die?" was his quick query. Nobody ever had asked me that before. "No, Gabe," I answered. "I don't think so." That prompted Gabe's follow-up. "Will we still get our Hanukkah and Christmas presents?" Good question. "You bet, Gabe."

The three kids were fine. Children want to know what is going on. Silence, the traditional answer my generation grew up on, would hurt more than would the truth. Colon cancer came and went, and the children took their cues from us. We avoided no cancer conversation with any of them but obviously were not stuck on the subject. And calm returned.

When the second cancer diagnosis came, life in our house was immediately different. Any suggestion of that old casual attitude was gone and forgotten. Meredith and I were shocked by the news. This was not supposed to happen. We said nothing for a while as the news settled in and composure returned.

Soon enough, we took our tested low-key approach with our kids, telling them that the doctor had not gotten all of the cancer and that sometimes this just happened. Certainly, we never mentioned the fear of liver involvement, which was discounted within days. The likely complications from the abdominal surgery were too complicated to go into with the kids. And we waited.

The surgeon was not available for a few weeks, and Meredith and I spent as much time at home as we could. And the clock just ticked. I coped with the written word, writing my personal manifesto about coping with MS and colon cancer for *The New York Times*. The final words in the article were "I will be fine." The piece was published on the day of the surgery. The kids smiled.

They weren't smiling when Meredith brought them to the hospital to visit. The morphine was potent, and my memory is vague. Gabe arrived and would not stay in the room. He saw the tubes, the IVs, and fled to the halls. There, blessed anonymity replaced intimacy and he seemed to feel safer. "It's so hard to see your parent sick with a sickness that kills people," Gabriel told me later, adding, "I was angry." So was I. Gabe should not have been put in that position, but he had insisted on coming. Choices for parents are tough. That scene was painful for all of us. I hated the thought of my kids seeing me in such a compromised state. Ben and Lily did not know what to say when they were in the room. I was too strung out on painkillers to say much of anything.

Home always offered an opportunity to normalize family contact, to draw the kids out on safe ground and take stock of their reactions and feelings. Life did change when Dad returned shortly after Thanksgiving after his second prizefight with colon cancer. The old man had gotten knocked around badly and was bruised and bloody when he came back from the hospital. I was in pain and decorated with that hated bag on my belly. The chill of late autumn had moved indoors.

Gray skies broke out each morning. I could not help it; in fact, I did not even realize what was happening. Bringing the emotion home from the wars was a stealth operation. The anger swept in beneath the radar and crawled into bed under the cover of my intense darkness. I could not detect the oozing bile, although everyone in the house knew it was there. My life was not supposed to have gone this way, and fear for the future was burning me up. I thought I was calm.

My head was down, and I was not seeing the people around me. Even slumped, I seemed to be casting glances over the heads of my children. I had assumed the kids would rejoice in my presence. They did not, instead shrinking from me in horror. My fangs were bared, and they were sharp. "Do your homework. Turn off the music," I snarled. "Clean up that mess," I commanded. "Don't leave it for your mother and me." I sat sullenly and stared, checking my watch in the evening so that I could order them to bed at precisely the appointed hour.

I was trapped in my own despair, uncomfortable and uncertain that I would mend. My colon was uncontrollable. The evidence was obvious to all around me. There were children spread evenly around the house. Those kids saw just about everything. What the children did not notice, they smelled. There is no humiliation quite like hearing one of your kids suggest a change of clothing. Roles were being reversed. My shame ran even deeper.

Self-conscious self-absorption became the by-product of illness. Bringing the furies to heel was impossible because their presence went unnoticed. My oblivion was complete, my psychotic behavior obvious to all but me. Deep inside myself I hid, cut off from family and friends. I left the cave only when summoned.

Finally my good wife had enough and sat me down. "You are becoming a monster," she warned, kindly adjusting her remarks to the present tense. My stare was blank. My emotional equilibrium is fine, I thought. What is she talking about?

Neither the warning nor the fact that my children walked around me dented the armor. I had felt them distancing themselves from me, in self-defense, no doubt. Lily would walk by me in a room and look the other way. "Open your eyes, Richard," my wife pleaded. "Don't do this to your children. You are not in this alone." I knew she was right. The beast had me by the neck. Escape was not easy. Anger is hard to legislate. The fires keep burning, the flames rising up regularly. Getting a grip became a long haul.

I decided to talk to the kids. We set the event as an interview. "Ben, you are thirteen. You can tell me the truth," I said quietly. "Have I been hard to live with?" Ben smiled suspiciously and sat, just staring at me. "Do you really want the truth?" he asked. I nodded, and the floodgates opened. "You were really mean," he began, pleased to unload and picking up steam.

"I wanted to scream in your face and kick

you," he added, "but Mom told me to cut you some slack." The smile on my face was gone. These were sobering statements. Gabe saw my blood flowing under the door and came in with his two cents. "It sounded like you really hate us." Lily wagged her finger in silence.

Pure pain had been dumped at my feet. Words would not come. A changed landscape would require more than words, anyway. The epiphany had hit hard. I had been so self-absorbed, and there was a lot more to think about than me. We patients do not lie alone in hospital beds. Our families are next to us, whether we see them or not.

The sun shone bright, the sky was particularly blue one late winter morning when I awoke to realize that I felt slightly better. Such observation becomes epiphany when the heavens have seemed dark for so long. The lack of light at tunnel's end had been difficult. On this morning I made coffee for Meredith and offered the kids pancakes. "Well, you're in a good mood," my good wife said dryly. I just looked at her. "Do you even realize how you have been treating us?" she asked. My stare was silent.

"You don't inflict your problems on

others," my dad has instructed me. Of course you don't, except you do, at least, I do. Perhaps it is inevitable. I am not a perfect person, and I was not able to stop myself from dropping my baggage on the toes of those I love the most. The old man is correct, of course, but when crisis comes, it is damned difficult actually to live by those words. A lot of slack must be cut in a family.

The kids seem to pay an emotional price two times, first dealing with my illnesses and then me. Their fears or fantasies about the future, the dark scenarios that invade young minds dealing with the illness of a parent must be intense. To compound that ordeal with my selfish anger only added to their burden.

What's next? At my house, somewhere in the back of small minds, I know that question silently lurks. As my children have watched me negotiate bad times, the anxiety on their faces betrays more than their concern for their dad. Unspoken but obvious, they have to wonder about their own lives.

Ben skates away from the subject. "You learn to cope with it," he says calmly. "You just do." Ben parrots his parents. How many times has Ben heard those words from us? I worry that his casual tone belies deep fears. "I do not believe it is going to happen to me.

I just don't," Ben says calmly. Denial may be in his genes. The dodge may have been learned at my knee and instinctively adopted. Maybe both. The warmth of blind security is comfortable, in fact seductive. But Ben does make a thoughtful point that anybody with a long-term health problem would do well to file fear in the drawer. "You can't keep thinking about stuff," he tells me. The world must offer kids a statute of limitations on the consuming concern and hurt. "Your sicknesses used to be a big thing to me," Ben says. "Now I am used to it. I think we all learn to just live."

The young person living with illness in a family and dealing with any disease that may be his or hers someday faces threats and challenges that probably will last a lifetime. The prospect of joining the family MS club must be frightening. Perhaps the assurances I hear from my children, their confidence in life and in themselves, are bravado.

Or perhaps they have grown stronger from the struggle. Our kids have been taught, if by example, to hang on to optimism. They do not fear their futures. They know they are loved. Whenever Meredith and I can find safe passage, they will be guided past pain. Embracing them is the most important act in our lives. The hugs come daily. "You know what, Lily?" I will ask. "Yeah. I know. You love me," she says in a conspicuously weary voice, finishing my sentence with a pronounced roll of the eyes. Her dramatics aside, Lily just may like hearing that. Expressions of love seem to cure some ills.

A young person facing the prospect of serious illness becomes a man-child, sometimes stripped of any childhood at all. We will not allow that to happen in our home. A child can develop a full appreciation for possibility and consequence just by growing up. That sensitivity, that intangible ability to understand is already apparent in our boys. Our kids seem to think, really to believe, that the world will not crumble for them under the weight of any circumstance.

My children ask questions touching on my health with no intention of hearing the answers, barely listening, it would seem, then abruptly changing the subject. My messages, the reassurances, must be received in some way, on some level, through those young ears. Maybe they want me to know that they care. Perhaps they just want to keep the subject alive.

"Lily, can we talk?" I asked one night. "I want to read," she answered. "Let me ask you something," I said softly. "It has been a while since the operations, since I was sick. I feel much better." "That's nice," Lily interrupted, perhaps uncomfortably. "Do you think things are better now?" I continued. Lily looked away and thought, though only for a moment. "It is better," she whispered. "Sort of." She laughed, adding, "Maybe." I smiled in silence. "You think you are pretty funny, don't you?" I finally asked. There was a pause. "Actually, I think you are funny," she answered with a straight face, "looking," she added. Lily sure knows how to deflect questions she would rather not face directly.

Smiling your way through sickness is a preposterous plan, though it can work wonders from time to time. My rose-colored glasses went into a drawer long ago. They are gathering dust, lying next to Meredith's cracked lenses of the same hue. Meredith had to discard dreams too soon in her life. She cannot have bargained for a relationship so defined by diseases. But that is what she got.

twelve

Meredith

When Meredith learned in the spring of 2002 that *Ladies' Home Journal* was planning another cover story about her for the following September, the black humor around our kitchen table ignited spontaneously. I started the pointed jokes about being cast as Richard, the house cripple. Meredith likes *LHJ*, but she half joined in. I could smell tragedy in the oven, just baking away.

Here we go again was all I could think. An *LHJ* cover story in October 2000 had been a sob story, the tale of the rising star and her crumpling husband, portraying me as physically devastated and Meredith as all-suffering. The magazine's cover and index chose the words "heartbreaking" and "devastating" to highlight my condition. Neither applied.

"Meredith Vieira's tears begin without

warning," the magazine wrote back then. That was the opening line. The tears are real and occasionally present in our house. Meredith has her emotional threshold, frequently different from mine. The tears are tempered with strength, however, and to lead this article with this maudlin suggestion that Meredith is only a weeping willow is misleading. Meredith can be one tough broad.

Now I was certain I would be portrayed in this next profile as even more of a wreck. Colon cancer had struck again, and I had written a series of very candid, personal essays in *The New York Times* about my health struggles, so I had already gone public. Meredith's life would be presented as even more of a soap opera. I did not like what I saw coming. "You should pose for the cover, sitting, perched on the arm of a wheelchair," I suggested. "Or maybe you should lie next to me in an oxygen tent." Meredith had a better idea. "How about if I just get out that cute little black dress I bought for your funeral, you know, just before the cancer surgery," she offered with a giggle. "I was so disappointed I never got to wear it."

My pessimistic scenario did not play out. The article was okay, only because Meredith headed off the martyr mania at the pass. I happened to call Meredith on her cellphone while she was lunching with the writer for the *Journal* piece. "Yeah, I am being interviewed," Meredith is quoted in the article as saying to me. "I am just at the part when I say I have to take care of you because you're a shadow of a man." Notes the interviewer, "My terminally pleasant interviewer's face freezes into what I suspect is a gargoyle-like grimace." I believe she got the point.

The September 2002 article was titled "What I Did for Love," suggesting that Meredith handed over the brass ring, compromising on career opportunities to tend to her ailing husband and family. She would have, I am sure, but that was not part of the plan. Meredith has done precisely what she has wished to do in her career. Her choices were about what gave her satisfaction. Meredith loves her work.

Our soggy drama has been a feature of the celebrity press for years. *The Star*, the rag sheet of record, started it off, crying about the "Secret Family Tragedy of TV Host Meredith Vieira" and revealing, sadly, of course, "Beautiful TV host Meredith Vieira hides a heartbreaking secret." That secret would be MS and me.

After my first bout with cancer, the floodgates opened wide. *TV Guide* carried a story labeling my wife "Super Meredith," who does it all because her husband is so sick. And *More* revised Meredith's history altogether: "Concerned about [Richard's] failing eyesight and coordination, she went from *60 Minutes* to a stint anchoring the *CBS Morning News*." Excuse me? Meredith was thrown overboard at *60 Minutes* because she was pregnant a second time and the old boys were already tired of hearing about Meredith and her new boy, with another on the way.

Ailing Richard is the public persona, my place in the annals of popular culture that my kids take in on some level. Even as I struggle to be a strong male role model and teach tough lessons about resolve and perseverance, these publications insist on presenting me as languishing somewhere between compromised and helpless. Do my children believe it? Some of the nonsense may rub off, and that makes my job with my kids that much harder. Also, it is infuriating.

Over the years I have become inured to our designated roles, Meredith the martyr and Richard the wretched, a burden she must bear on her back. It is a version of our lives made to order for slick articles in the tabloids and women's magazines, but it is not the truth, which is much more complex and textured. Here is the real story.

We are happy people. We laugh a lot. Meredith and I are quirky people who get by with a little help from our friends. Vieira and Cohen are not the all-American types. The Cleavers would never invite them to supper. Nobody much does. Meredith and I tend to keep to ourselves, not because of sickness but because we can be reclusive, and we like to hang out with each other and our kids.

We are quite ordinary, though, and we do it our way. We do not watch much television or go to football games. We own vans and drive them into the ground. I dislike hot dogs and marching bands. I hate to shave. Meredith hates wearing underwear, which she never misses the opportunity to tell America from her perch on *The View* (she neglects to add that she does wear ratty old leotards under those fancy clothes). And Meredith does not like answering telephones, often refusing to respond to the ringing, even when she is next to the instrument as it is screaming.

Our idea of a good time is to gather with friends at our house and hold court, drinking too much wine and talking late into the night. We enjoy our close friends, and we are a tight family. There are no martyrs living on any floor of our house. Martyrs are not welcome. Laughter is, and happy noises are commonly heard exploding out of open windows. So is the blissful sound of children fighting. Shrieks of despair are a fiction. We do not come home in the evenings to solemnly light candles and mourn.

Yet it would be a lie to say that my illness has not forced major changes in the way Meredith and I interact, in the way we see each other, and in the way we feel about each other. Sickness does overtake and take over lives and it has exacted a precious toll on our relationship. Our partnership has been buffeted, altered in a long evolution of pressures and reactions to health crises, fallout that continues. The book of our lives is being rewritten in sometimes painful ways, as the core of a relationship we cherish shifts and groans under the weight of stress and uncertainty. It is a far different relationship than it was at the beginning.

When Meredith visited me on Cape Cod in 1983, we were still getting to know each other. Our relationship was exciting, our mutual attraction warming as rapidly as the dunes leading down to the sea in the August sun. Meredith and I walked around Provincetown and sat to talk, drank wine, and watched glowing sunsets. We played endless games of chess; Meredith tried to cheat rather than lose. We bought lobsters to prepare for dinner one evening, but Meredith suddenly decided that they must be liberated, their claws freed, the gawky red bottom crawlers returned to the sea.

For Meredith, this gesture took on a magical significance. I only shrugged, watching twenty-five dollars floating off to Portugal. At that moment, though, I knew Meredith was serious and I was hooked. Meredith had already stopped calling me Rich. Now it was Richard. The small signals speak the story. I gave her a ratty old stuffed lobster I found on the back of a shelf at my parents' house. Meredith was to take the cloth crustacean home to Chicago. "Free it in Lake Michigan," I told her. Our futures seemed tied together.

I had few specific expectations, only the fantasy of a straightforward, uncomplicated relationship. Of course, my life was already growing complex and Meredith was about the most complicated person I could have chosen to hit head-on. Meredith can be volatile. The woman also can be disarming. "You know how insecure I am," she tells me from time to time. Meredith used to be delightfully unsure of herself. Then she became a talk show host and now knows everything.

I wanted my health not to be an issue. Desperately. But multiple sclerosis would have to be a factor in the relationship. There was no way around that. Truth in advertising demanded an honest accounting for health. How illness would play was unknown. "I knew you had MS," Meredith says, "but I imagined the best and did not think about the worst." Reality was our professional game but not a personal strength. Meredith and I did not appreciate the inevitability of physical change for the worst. "Your progress seemed quite slow," she tells me. "It never seemed real. I knew it was, but you cannot plan for what might happen," Meredith adds.

Meredith showed no discomfort with my multiple sclerosis, though it was a common topic of conversation, usually raised by me. "I just stopped thinking about the whole thing," Meredith admits. "The discussion was not going anywhere. There was nothing that could be resolved. You seemed so healthy. I made myself believe that would always be the case."

The talk of illness slowly fell away. We kept moving, forward, as if by plan. And we stayed in motion. "You were somebody who liked to go out and just walk around the city for hours. Do you remember that?"

Meredith asks. "That was your idea of a date. Once, we took the Staten Island Ferry and walked to midtown. You must remember that. Oy. You were so weird. You had a strange idea of a date."

We did walk, and we ran. We ran, then ran some more, on beaches and back roads, in Manhattan's Riverside Park, Chicago's Lincoln Park, and in foreign lands. Running was the common denominator, our great leveler. Meredith ran faster than I could. I ran longer distances than she would. We competed, though the race seemed never to be against each other. We ran against ourselves, trying always to be faster and stronger.

Running forged an equality that became a symbol for us, the action photograph of our very essence, who we were and how we wanted to live. Meredith seemed to be running toward something, I away. "It was as if you could outrun your problems," Meredith told me years later.

I could not, though. Eventually compromised health forced me off the running paths. Meredith clearly longs for that past, our brand of shared adventure. Her eyes grow sad just talking about our active life together. "Running together and hiking up mountains were very important to me, to us," Meredith says. "They were something we could have shared with the kids."

That is a true source of disappointment for us both, an experience I will not share with any child of mine. I watch Ben ascend a hill at steady speed, sometimes with his mom. I long to be there. The loss of our multiyear marathon conjures up a different kind of photograph in Meredith's album, the snapshot of reality tinged with bitterness. "Sometimes you talk about being diminished. I am diminished, too," Meredith says. "It would be wonderful if you could be an equal."

The statement is fair. We no longer are equals. That admission is offered with pain, even on paper. Hearing the doubt expressed, the sheer frustration of my partner, the questioning of a relationship built on a common view of equal status undermines my fundamental sense of self. Meredith has every right to feel that way. The sense of equality I once derived from running has been replaced by biting feelings of inadequacy.

"Sometimes I feel you are my fourth child," Meredith says with a small glint of humor, though the remark is not funny at all. The statement validates what I have long felt. My hands do not work. Meredith must button my cuffs, sometimes put the key in the lock and turn it. My eyes do not work. She must find the pencil I have dropped, measure the pancake mix. "Your physical needs can be overwhelming," Meredith tells me. Wife to mother is a sad transition.

I watched my parents exchange roles long ago, my mother having to take charge as my dad's body failed. My mind conjures up images of my mother, always there at my father's side. She stands by him, always watching, arms ready to steady the old man as he moves. My dad is always unsteady, frequently looking as if he will fall at any moment. My mother is a nurturing soul. My father is the old man. She is Mom. She takes his elbow as he steps gingerly onto a curb or climbs a few stairs.

Meredith has taken to making those same protective gestures to me. The moves are subtle, almost unconscious on her part. Even when Meredith is engaged in conversation with someone else, her radar is turning. She just shows up at critical moments, looking away, paying no attention, and watching me like a hawk. Hovering is an acquired skill.

It used to be so different. We had been equals, personally and professionally. Meredith was a correspondent before the camera; I a producer behind the scenes and invisible. Meredith sat on a throne; I became a power behind it. I was making more money than Meredith, an accident of history that we knew would soon change. But neither of us was counting dollars or notches on our belts. Meredith and I felt good about our shared opportunities and power, about ourselves, and about us. We loved our lives.

That began to change when I began to fall. There had been numbness here, an evolving limp there, making falls inevitable. They came, and that's when my strong self-esteem, my bulletproof shield, began to crack. The little accidents, short drops, and hard landings ended on safe enough ground. But the quick stumbles and tumbles added up, bringing the humiliation of public weakness. What is this kid doing on the street alone? I thought to myself about myself.

The self-doubt rubbed off on my marriage and became doubt about me. "I did begin to see you differently when you started falling," Meredith says. "You would leave the house, and stuff would happen. You were so upset when you came home. I began to worry more." What Meredith will not say is that she was losing confidence in my ability to function on my own and without consequence.

In my head I saw Meredith stepping away. The more I questioned my abilities, the greater became my hesitation to go forth and succeed. And the more unattractive I felt. My motivation to engage professionally declined and radiated palpable weakness. Projecting a lack of strength is not good in a marriage or in any intimate relationship. Who wants to embrace a bowl of Jell-O? I, and I think Meredith, felt distance between us.

The imbalance between Meredith and me, the widening gap in our self-confidence and self-esteem, was marked. By the mid-1990s, Meredith's career with *The View* was exploding upward while I had realized that a conventional job, any regular work, was probably physically out of reach. My bitterness festered quietly, obvious only to my wife, whose only crime was roaring success.

I did not begrudge Meredith her hard-won ascent, but our relationship was radically altered. Responsibilities changed, roles reversed. A lopsided power structure evolved in our house. Meredith and I never had subscribed to traditional expectations or conventional notions of what roles men and women should play in the high drama of marriage, but the changes hit me hard.

Neither Meredith nor I was driven by money, ever. We both had made enough money to live as we chose. Financial responsibilities were not an issue until children arrived, with the need for us to plan for their futures. Meredith worked in front of the camera, and her income had long eclipsed mine. "How does it feel to have your wife making so much more than you?" friends and acquaintances would wonder out loud. Some actually asked in just those words. "I feel humiliated," I answered, "all the way to the bank." Still, the wide disparity in what we brought home did feed feelings of not doing enough. Something was amiss when I could not afford a pork chop and Meredith was bringing home so much bacon.

Meredith is doing what she wants to do, I told myself, not because she has to. "Everyone wants to be taken care of," Meredith counters to me. "I wish I never had to work. You never believe me, but it's true." Those words are hard to hear. "Of course, if I had that life," she adds, "I probably would want a career." Meredith laughs, but she sees her life both ways. "You would be bored if you just stayed home," I tell her. "Try me," she responds. Meredith loves what she does more than she will admit, though. Quit? I do not picture Meredith staying home, startling the cat with news of her wardrobe while the kids are in school.

Push comes to shove only with the endless rigor and routine of raising our kids. The suburbs are spread out, and we must travel by car. I am relegated to passenger status, forever riding shotgun. Because Meredith wears the wings, occupying the driver's seat, we just see each other differently. That imbalance is an example of what slowly redefines a relationship.

Sometimes I am not in the car at all. It is easier to stay home. I sit on the porch, staying home with one kid or other, sipping tequila and reading a biography, while Meredith spends her evenings touring a large county, driving carloads of kids to weekend parties, then killing time, waiting to pick them back up. She buys birthday presents and juggles schedules, hopscotching neighborhoods to deliver kids to events, always barely in the nick of time.

"I wish you could drive," Meredith says to me in exasperation. "I cannot, Meredith," my hypercalm answer always comes. "I know you can't, Richard," she concedes apologetically. "I just wish you could." Right. "So do I," comes the last word. This is our ritual. Meet Sisyphus and his rock. I would gladly trade that bottle and book for a set of car keys. Meredith hates to drive. I love the road. A car would mean freedom. All I want, someday, if but once, is to slip into that front seat again, driver's side, to stretch out behind the wheel, push the clutch to the floor, shift, and go.

I am a problem, and in my worst moments I think I should go. But I have a family and will not. Here I remain. I just keep my perspective and remember what is important. My failing eyesight and clumsy fingers put the thousand small tasks of parenting and partnering out of reach. We live with that, too. Meredith suffers in the silence of one who is used to the drill. Though I never get used to the scene, it seems second nature to her by now.

Blunt questions to Meredith about dreams, disappointments, and regrets elicit blank looks and shrugs. "It is what it is, Richard," she says without emotion, adding, "I find picking this stuff apart very self-indulgent. You cannot predict anything in life. Do I wish we could go back even three or four years? Sure."

That period of our lives, three or four years ago, before cancer, marks a demarcation zone, the end of relative calm and the beginning of major trouble. Before cancer, we had found a rhythm to our existence. Whatever the frustrations, the MS miseries and struggles, we seemed to have made our peace with our lives. For my many limitations, I offered stability and shared a brand of common sense that contributed to the lives of my family.

Colon cancer changed everything. "The cancer," Meredith says with a grimace. "Whoa. Out of nowhere. Twice." She stops. "This was going to be serious. I knew it." Colon cancer had come from nowhere, roaring around the bend like a fast last lap at Indy. The disease knocked us over and kicked us hard.

Meredith forgets the worst or has a marvelous capacity for forgiveness. "You are loved in this home, Richard," Meredith tells me. "I love you. The kids love you." A pause. The lady chuckles. "We just cannot stand being around you." Everyone is a comedian. Laughter comes often, though sometimes self-consciously. We do not always find it easy to lighten up.

We are not different from families across America struggling with illness. Our bags are a little heavier, perhaps, our heads higher in the clouds. As a family, we struggle to have it all. Meredith can feel very alone. "You are a dreamer," she tells me. "I make the trains run on time," she says, pointing to the logistical nightmare of parenting, the relentless attention to helping children across the minefields before them. "You are the one who is sick. You have paid a terrible price. I just want to keep the kids emotionally healthy."

That is the bottom line of our lives, and Meredith struggles to remain in one piece emotionally. "I used to be an optimist," Meredith says. "Life would be better tomorrow than today. I believed that. I was a happy person, you know, almost carefree. I'm afraid that is gone," Meredith says in a firm, resolute voice.

We were all almost carefree once. We clung to the idea of life as adventure for a long time. Our twenties and even our thirties knew big opportunity and little pain. Then we had to grow up when the bill came due. Nothing impinges on a life without care like a mortgage and a few children. Illness is only the unfortunate icing on the cake.

Too often, the physical and emotional pain of illness is visited on spouses and children. That is a regrettable truth that applies to us. If coping is a family activity, my wife and kids can claim a large stake. They, too, are victims. We wear the same clothes and eat the same food. In many ways, we are the same person. My family's burden is equal to mine. For Meredith that is especially true. Cancer and multiple sclerosis have pulled the rug from under me, but she knows she is the one who must remain standing.

Standing becomes a euphemism for guarding the emotional health and equilibrium of others, holding it all together. Meredith joins Atlas with the feeling of a world on her shoulders. If she would lighten up, she would notice how brightly the sun shines on her world. "We do have a good life," Meredith admits. "I look around at what we have built. Our kids. And I do feel grateful."

And I am grateful to her. Meredith is there for us. She provides the glue in our family. Embracing others is her avocation. It does not take a red light on a camera for Meredith to be on. She is always on. "I feel tired. All of the time," Meredith sighs. "I know this sounds self-important," she adds, "but I am nervous that if something happens to me, something bad . . ." Meredith goes silent for a moment. "I am scared everything will fall apart."

If there is anything Meredith teaches by example, it is survival.

thirteen

A Resilient Man

The trudge from the train promised to become a vertical climb on this sweltering summer day. The hill, a suburban Mount Everest to a disabled guy having a bad day, looked formidable as it reached for the sky. The late afternoon summer sun was scorching, temperatures pressing one hundred degrees and climbing. Soon, much to my dismay, I would be doing the same.

My phone calls home from the clattering train had become 911 pleas, with no answer at the other end. The endless rings at the house meant no ride up the hill from the station. The Hudson was still as I stepped off the train, wavy lines of heat like ribbon candy, rising into the haze above the tiny whitecaps dotting the river.

Heat is the enemy of MS, as Gabe and I

painfully had been reminded only a year earlier. I assured myself that I felt strong, and things would be easier this time. They never are, but the hope remains. The climb up zigzagging streets and paths began. Soon I was dragging my feet and tripping along, veering side to side as much as up, my equilibrium short-circuiting in a cascading sweat. I was struggling to stay on my feet. My right arm could no longer summon the strength to carry my sport jacket. I needed my left hand for the cane, so the coat had to go back on my dripping frame.

Cars sped past as I kept climbing, swaying and staggering like a drunk. In a town where people routinely help each other, drivers stared blankly out their windows and silently kept going. Who picks up drunks? I made frequent stops to rest, leaning against parked cars, holding on to trees or any inanimate objects that would have me. When I walked straight into a telephone pole, the collision came in slow motion, my gait so slow that the impact was barely felt.

Finally, I hit the house, staggering, backpack and jacket falling to the ground outside the front door. This sweaty struggle was all too familiar, the day's trek only the latest reminder of how high life's hills can be. But the pain of the ordeal was more emotional than physical. A vague anger, bordering on self-loathing, washes over me in these compromised situations. Once again, my bumbling weakness was pushed into my face. I was a child again. Surely I must be to blame for not getting up the hill more gracefully. Somewhere inside, I felt the anguish was deserved. There is an anger at myself that will not go away.

Of course, this poisoned reaction makes no sense. My illnesses were thrust on me, not ordered by mail from the L. L. Bean catalog. I do feel like less of a person, though. Perhaps I turn the anger against myself because there are no other available targets in sight and I simply cannot accept what I have become.

A diminished man lives upstairs at my house.

This fellow struggles each day to see beyond what has been taken, to view himself for what remains and to celebrate what he still can accomplish in his life. The final battle of illness is for the high ground of emotional health, to accept limitations and pursue the dream of a successful life. More succinctly, my crusade is to make peace with myself.

The quest for that peace has become an endless search for self-esteem. It is a dangerous expedition, crossing innumerable emotional minefields. The enemy is me, and I am watching. Finding my way is measured in the distance between once high expectations for my life and the powerful, cold reality of the day. This is a time of reckoning, a hard-nosed assessment of my life.

"Meredith, I just cannot do that anymore" has become my all-too-frequent mantra when confronting a physical challenge I used to take for granted. Putting on my socks has become a tiring journey. With upsetting frequency, I am forced to admit that my limitations are only increasing, with no end in sight.

My long march is reflected in the eyes of my children, the arms of my wife. I am not in this alone. Loved ones map my life because our journey is taken together. Objectives are no clearer than feeling better about myself tomorrow than I do today, and moving forward in the direction I charted for myself so many years ago.

Making my peace and seeing that level of comfort mirrored in those who matter the most are what the journey is all about. My family takes its cues from me. They hover and observe. The kids instinctively adjust their view of our relationship to perceptions of how Dad feels about them, usually meaning how their old man feels about himself. My level of self-esteem varies according to the frustrations of the moment.

A man of severe limitations shares space at our house. He is saddened by the disappointments of his life, buoyed by his successes. This man creeps around the top floor like the madman of the movies, the wild-eyed guy with the crazy hair. As a creature of my mind's eye, I try to be introspective, too often judging myself harshly. I want to do more, and I feel like a mutant. And I hurt.

These are private thoughts that rarely spill over in view of others. They do exist, however, and the feeling of inadequacy is powerful. "Are you ever embarrassed being seen with me?" I asked Meredith in frustration one day. "Yes," she answered quickly, "but not for the reasons you think." No laugh was audible. "You have got to get over this thing you have about yourself," she added.

Easier said than done. The hurt runs so deep. I hurt myself physically every day. These are the small injuries of someone no longer in control of his body: catching a finger in a window, tripping up the stairs, stumbling into the vertical edge of a doorway. I fall on my face with the best of them, feeling sharp pain from each predictable mishap. The emotional pain feels much worse. My scream is silent, but it reverberates in my ears for minutes. Can you fucking believe this? I demand to know of no one in particular. Can you believe *I* did this to myself?

The sense of being beaten down cannot be coaxed out of me and banished. The timbre of my body has softened. Too often I slump, looking down instead of peering up into the distance. I feel weak because I acknowledge the realities of my life. We exist in a culture that celebrates strength. Men are strong and self-reliant. I am weakened and need the help of others. There is no escape from the rust I see on my body.

I must rise above the culture of perfection and remember that I can *be* even if I can no longer *do*. I am learning to acknowledge weakness, accept assistance, and discover new forms of self-definition. My formula has changed. I do not read self-absorbed men's magazines or go to Vin Diesel movies. A new male ideal will have to do and might even save me. I will just have to create it. I cannot allow myself to be held captive by old dreams.

Success today comes by a different standard, measured by more cerebral achievements and often centered on the lives of my children. Those kids *are* the center of my life. Careers evolve into jobs, and sooner or later it becomes apparent to most of us that there is a lot more to life than professional recognition. Dealing with challenges to health is a great ally in nurturing that change in priorities.

Seeing the suffering that comes from illness — and it is all around me — has changed me. It has softened me, though Meredith might not believe that. What I want my children to learn has come into sharp relief. I want them to become good and sensitive adults, to recognize that they are more fortunate than many. And they are on their way.

My kids watch over me. Having had to be concerned for another at a tender age, they have had to abandon the narcissism of youth. That is not all bad. "Be careful, Dad," Gabe warns. "Don't trip over those roots." We have wandered off the sidewalk, and he is worried for me. We take our kids and their friends to a movie. The show is in one of New York's vertical multiplex monstrosities. The endless escalator rides carry us high. The crowds are crushing. As each escalator expedition approaches a new floor, Gabe turns and yells through the packed bodies and din, "Be careful, Dad. We're at the end again. Don't fall."

As with most parents, I used to think only of caring for my own. A young child looking out for a parent seemed to go against the natural order of things. That view has changed. Love from a child plays out with warm, meaningful gestures. My children are learning important lessons about life. That people are not perfect. That some of us need help. These lessons are worthwhile.

I struggle to move beyond the guilt that my children must live with my problems. My kids are wonderful friends, and when they do come to my aid, I am getting better at dismissing the remorse I feel about not being able to be the caretaker.

Everyone in the house but the dog is in the act. We stand in the kitchen at our house. "Richard, I'll do that," Meredith says, moving in swiftly after hearing the shattering glass and reaching for the broom. "You can't see well enough." I cringe in silence. We drive down the street. "Why don't you wait in the car," Meredith suggests as she jumps out to finish a few errands I should be sharing. "I will just be a minute." I wait. Ben and I amble through town. "Dad, there's a bench," Ben points out on a local street. "Hang out there, okay? The store is a long walk. I will be right back." And I sit.

These are scenes from my life. I am the beleaguered character feeling small next to the beautiful leading lady who has grown larger than life. Continuous compromise takes a cumulative toll, the body in motion, now at rest and likely to remain so. This is not the sporadic choreography of the occasional bad weekend, a one-time twisted ankle or sore knee. Standing on the sidelines is a way of life. The psychological fallout only adds up and multiplies, weighing heavy.

A stronger man than he knows walks down the stairs each day at my house. I have survived thirty years of a war with my body and countless battles with my psyche. Resignation presides. So does resolve. Personal strength, in the end, wins out. My hope never dies. And, still, I call myself an optimist. I believe that in the end, my life will be better. That is why I can still get up the hill in the heat.

The diminished man must find a way to live, though stripped of his power. He needs perspective. What once was an imperative must be replaced by objectives of higher value. The journalist sprinting through foreign streets crowded with humanity is missed but no longer so important. The giggling child daring his dad to tag him when legs are not strong enough for the chase is of greater consequence.

"Watch me, Ben," I now cry out silently in a waking dream. Hold the bat this way, I think as I watch a boy learn for himself what I can no longer show him. I long to be a powerful, masculine role model, partly from my innate narcissism, but more to be the role model I enjoyed as a child. My old man was everything I wanted him to be. (My dad's disease had showed up after I was out of the house.) I am only what my children must wish I could be.

The dream of being the undaunted, indestructible dad dies hard: the power flickers, returning in my mind's eye for a moment. I fly down the stairs early one morning, stopping to slide into a seat in the den, threading a needle and hurriedly sewing a button back onto my dress shirt. Quickly, the wrinkled shirt is stowed in my gym bag. I am on the run.

Hurriedly finishing my coffee, I yell back upstairs to one of my sons, telling him to grab his tennis racquet and hurry along so we can get going. Get the car keys, I remember. Hurry, I cajole this young man, still slowly waking. My meeting is in one hour. We want to play a set. I jump into the car. The machine roars. I push the clutch with a strong left leg, shift, and we are gone. The fantasy is painful self-indulgence. Desire runs deep but goes nowhere.

Frustration mixes with sadness for what my children and I each miss, the vital companionship of a father and children sharing a common passion for the active life. The boys had chosen sports, Lily the stage. The awful sense of betraying my children's dreams is acute. Can my kids look up to a man looking down? Others say it is all in my head. As children go about their business, they seem to see only a father, a man who loves them. They may not even know the concept of a diminished man or think in those terms.

My children know what I can no longer do. I have no reason to believe my weakness is judged harshly, except, of course, by my biggest critic. Me. When I throw a ball with the boys, the ball is slowly rolled back on the ground, where it can be seen. My weak right arm launches endless wild pitches that are forgiven and retrieved in good humor. The kids see it all and forgive just about everything. I cannot seem to do the same.

What tears at me is that surely I must appear to be flawed in the eyes of my children.

I do believe that what matters to them is that we play ball at all. The terms of the game do not matter. But surely they wish they had more. My kids are resilient because they see the same quality in their parents. Perhaps I am a role model in an arena that matters more than the field of play.

But I cannot stop feeling like a child. "Let's go to a movie," little Lily suggests. "We can take a cab," she adds, before I can remind her that I no longer drive. Dependence can be a dreadful by-product of disease, even if it is routine for others in the family.

When my children are grown and gone, what will they remember about living with me? Will the physical flaws of their father stick in their minds, because a sick parent may be an unforgettable sight, or will they choose to remember something much better? I worry that memory will zero in on the diminished man I think I have learned to recognize staring out from the mirror. The doubts and painful questions may not give my children enough credit. Perhaps my kids will forget to remember what I cannot put behind me. What I could not do may have less staying power than what I did.

Gabe is a child of touch, the physical embrace. When I tuck him into his bed at night, he will ask me to scratch his back and rub his legs. When he throws his arms around my neck and kisses me, he says quite simply, "I love you, Daddy." I know he has taken in more than my foibles and flaws on that day. Gabriel gets something from me. Somewhere inside, buried or hidden away on some level, my entire family must understand that the real person is not in the sneakers but in the soul. Why can't I settle that score for myself?

How diminished am I? Am I an incomplete person? *Diminished* is a subjective term, I know, resting in the eye of the beholder. My notion of the diminished body may not match yours. When John Patterson, a popular professor at Columbia, died in my first semester at the journalism school, Walter Cronkite offered a personal remembrance of their radio days together. Walter spoke glowingly of a man in a wheelchair. "John lost both legs, actually after World War Two," Cronkite said at a memorial service, "but he was not diminished." Walter paused. "John laid the lie to the old canard that those who can, do. Those who cannot, teach."

The ability to do still haunts me, though I try to teach myself that there are many routes to where I want to be. Patterson's legs were gone, lost in a fall under a train at war's end. The man had to chart a new course for himself. He found his future in a classroom, teaching graduate students to write for radio. I, too, have fallen into the safety net of more passive pursuits. They include teaching from time to time at Columbia, the very institution that offered John his own shelter.

I've learned that the great escape from physical flaws and the emotional vulnerability traveling not far behind is the mad dash into my own head. The recesses of my identity are dark and inviting. Privacy and peace are mine in that comfortable zone. Inventing your own reality can be a side trip worth taking, a respite from the harsher life on the outside. The fields of my mind are fertile. Cerebral skills are an equalizer of vast proportion.

My friend Cronkite sauntered into a men's room after the evening news one day long ago. The venerable anchor stood beside me at a urinal. We could have been sitting at the library or in a crowded theater. We were on equal footing. In the depths of my head, the weakened physical state does not matter. If I use my head, I can be whom I want, because I can count on my brain more than my body.

Then what does define a diminished person? Common culture creates male expectations that are conventional if not shallow. We like to beat our chests and cut notches on our belts. Strong muscles and clear vision, the ability to kick the ball a mile and push the pedal to the metal, seem too trivial to amount to much. A good life requires something more sensitive and special than that. Rising above the prosaic patterns of male life in America can be difficult, even for one who sees through the thin veneer of masculinity and recognizes the trap he cannot seem to stop falling into. We are but prisoners of the standard measure.

I want to believe that what I offer my children has value, that sensitivity and human decency teach their own lesson. Sharing a passion for history and music, teaching a kid to play Beethoven on his cheeks or list state capitals in a hurry, count for something. Acting as role model and showing grace and humor in the face of adversity mean more than driving a car. Being a good person must carry more gravitas than the ability to run, jump, and play. These are special qualities that have been sharpened by the pain of grievous illness. I am legally disabled but able to stand on my own.

I believe I am a better person for the journey I have been forced to take for these many years. Anyone can go seventy miles per hour in a fifty-five zone or beat another out for a taxi in the rain. My survival skills are strong but sensitivity flourishes. The world of television news is amply stocked with managers and anchors with small personal gyroscopes and large egos.

I might have been one of those people once. That certainly is where I was headed. I wonder what I would have become, living my ambitions in good health. Multiple sclerosis and cancer have proved to be tools of personal growth. Let me be clear. I would trade sickness for, say, a used car anytime. But I think back many years ago to the tired old tennis racquet, flung far in frustration because I did not have my way on the court. How immature I was, how grounded in the moment. I choose battles more selectively now. There is a more ordered view of what is important. Maybe, just maybe, I am a better parent.

Walking an elderly woman hobbling with a cane across a busy street recently was second nature, even as others rushed around her. I wished my kids were there. This is not about virtue or plaques for good citizenship. We all benefit from greater sensitivity toward others. I learned that lesson long ago and the hard way, to be sure. Disease adds dimension to a person, depth to the soul. In the end, that is not so bad.

"Lily, let me ask you something," I said as I sat on her bed to tuck her in one night. "Do you know what respect is?" Lily looked up from her book but said nothing. "Do you admire us?" I asked, trying to clarify my question. "You and Mom?" she asked. I nodded my head. "I admire Mom," she said with a small laugh. "You're chopped liver." Sometimes I take what I can get.

I had to smile at cutting humor. Those of us who battle chronic illness are in it for the long haul. I need to come to grips with who I am and what is important before I can function at my best with others. That has yet to happen, for I am a work in progress with no end in sight. Coping is forever an aspiration. I need to stop getting hung up on conventional issues of control and inabilities that just do not matter.

We all need to appreciate ourselves for what we are and stop whining about what we are not. I grow weary of wishing so desperately for something else. Those concerns find no resolution. All I can do is do what I can do, which is precious little. I am beginning to shed passivity and taking a more active role in my health. I even chose a new doctor who I knew would force me into a more active role.

"If you want to be treated here, you have to change," the neurologist directing a major MS research and treatment center in New York told me. "You have to get serious and get involved in your own care. We demand a lot from our patients."

The moment was sobering. A new era had to begin. Coping evolves. It was time to take charge and stop making a monkey of myself. There is work to be done. Trying to sneak away from the truth worked for a long time but now seemed foolish. Adulthood must be learned anew from time to time. The course of treatment is rigorous. The thought of three injections of interferon each week instead of one is daunting. "It's about time," Meredith said when I told her. "It makes sense to me." My body is there. I never know about my head.

There are no cures out there, and there can be no illusions of health getting better. I do dream of living something better. Constantly. That ethereal notion of a life remains undefined. There is peace of mind out there somewhere. That calm may take years to find, but its promise carries me beyond regions I otherwise would visit. To dream is to fly. I create my world and live in it.

Dreaming is rising above emotional pain, believing that life will be better, no matter what the physician decrees. Optimism may fly in the face of what the Greek chorus chants. So what? Let the soothsayers don sackcloth and ashes. I reach higher than the realities of my life. Self-doubt remains. So does determination.

Life sucks and then you die. So the cynic says. For some of us, that grim assessment of humanity's joint venture may prove true, but there is nothing to be gained by wallowing in disappointment. My big plans do not have to factor in reality. Frankly, they are not so big. I will not be training for the next Olympics. Pity. I have been running so hard for so long. I am in great shape.

A resilient man returns each night to my house.

This man knows his body will not halt the evolution downward, but he is determined. He is proud. He is a survivor who sees his own frailties and flaws, knows doubt and fear. This man yields to nothing. He sounds weak to himself and knows he is not. This man cannot win, but he knows he must not lose until the journey is done. Don Quixote had nothing over him in seeing challenges on his own terms. That is his virtue, a mysterious ability to define his own power and mission and pursue a dream, perhaps delusional, in the face of a reality he cannot accept.

"Our deepest fear is not that we are inadequate," Nelson Mandela tells us. "Our deepest fear is that we are powerful beyond measure. It is our light, not our darkness that most frightens us. . . . And as we let our light shine, we unconsciously give other people permission to do the same."

And so, I will continue living in my head. For me, fighting the war to cope and to live life my way continues, often around the clock. Thoughts of what in the world I am going to do tomorrow, how I am going to live today, stay in my mind, even in my dreams. Coping is a process that does not end. That job will not be completed until I have finished my journey, declaring victory in my final moments and heading for home.

In the quieter regions of my mind, the work goes on. The job of getting by continues long after the whistle signals the end of the workday. In my marvelous journeys into the night, I am working through the circumstances of my life, ever probing or imagining. Dreaming. The wheel turns, always. Images of a compromised life fill my head. I want to and try to rise above them. Whether that head is held high, eyes straight ahead, or I slump, my gaze sinking as I peer through fog to an uncertain future, my stride stays as strong as my body permits. There are miles to go, and I must stay in motion. I reach, and in my dreams I soar.

In the safety of my mind on one magic night, the warm breeze was embracing as I left earth on a shining morning. I ran down a gentle hill, legs sure, stretched forward and steady. My arms extended out as wings. I went aloft in the simplicity of perfect flight. Lifted gracefully above a flowered hill, my body was strong, my vision flawless, and I could see forever. At last the war was over. I gained altitude without effort. The grace of elegant motion was mine, and I was accepted forever into the billowy clouds.

About the Author

RICHARD M. COHEN is a former senior producer for CBS News and CNN, a three-time Emmy Award winner, and the recipient of numerous honors in journalism. He is a contributor to the "Health and Fitness" section of the *New York Times* and lives with his family outside New York City.

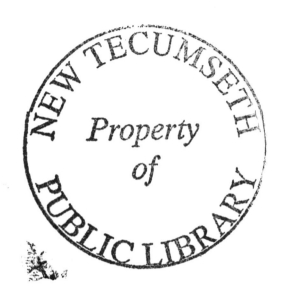